Craig White has .... he University of Gl... of Psychological Medicine at the same university. He has a doctor........ in clinical psychology from the University of Manchester and completed a postgraduate certificate in cognitive therapy at the University of Durham. He is a Founding Fellow of the Academy of Cognitive Therapy.

Craig has devoted his career to ensuring that NHS services are more responsive to people's psychological needs. This has been evident in his pioneering work recognizing the importance of changes in thinking following stoma surgery, resulting in his book *Living with a Stoma* (Sheldon Press, second edition 2010). It can also be seen in his work on understanding psychosocial adjustment to cancer and developing psychological care and therapies for people with physical illness, and his work with the Scottish Government on self-management.

More recently, he has championed person-centred approaches to the management of significant adverse events and handling of complaints in NHS Scotland. He has also developed a programme of research work focused on understanding how to improve supportive care approaches in cancer. His commitment to supporting evidence-based psychological care has been further demonstrated through writing this book on how best to manage complicated grief reactions effectively.

Overcoming Common Problems Series

Selected titles

A full list of titles is available from Sheldon Press,
36 Causton Street, London SW1P 4ST and on our website at
www.sheldonpress.co.uk

Overcoming Common Problems

Living with Complicated Grief

PROFESSOR CRAIG A. WHITE

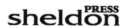
sheldon **PRESS**

First published in Great Britain in 2013

Sheldon Press
36 Causton Street
London SW1P 4ST
www.sheldonpress.co.uk

British Library Cataloguing-in-Publication Data
A catalogue record for this book is available from the British Library

ISBN 978-1-84709-150-5
eBook ISBN 978-1-84709-304-2

Typeset by Fakenham Prepress Solutions, Fakenham, Norfolk NR21 8NN
First printed in Great Britain by Ashford Colour Press
Subsequently digitally printed in Great Britain

Produced on paper from sustainable forests

To Gwen, Adam and Daniel, who have constantly sustained and supported me in my work

Contents

Acknowledgements

I am grateful to Fiona Marshall for commissioning this book, and particularly for her support and patience when distress made it difficult for me to focus on this work. Thank you to Phil Wong for expertly enabling and empowering me to complete this project. I would also like to acknowledge the work of Dr Katherine Shear who has pioneered the psychological treatment of complicated grief and whose treatment protocols have informed the self-help approach to managing complicated grief that I have outlined in this book. I would also like to acknowledge the people who have attended my clinics for help with complicated grief reactions and the staff of BMI Carrick Glen Hospital for their efficient support of my clinical practice during the time I have been writing this book. The families I have met in my work as Assistant Director at NHS Ayrshire and Arran have also provided helpful insights into traumatic bereavement and the way in which organizations can support and help when things go wrong. Sincere thanks are also due to my colleagues at NHS Ayrshire and Arran and the University of the West of Scotland for their support and encouragement.

Introduction

Acute, crushing grief after the loss of a loved one is normal. The process of making sense of a world that has dramatically changed after a bereavement is painful and distressing. The grief journey takes time, is often erratic and turbulent, and cannot be evaded. 'There is no way out of the desert except through it', as the African saying has it. And there is no going back, no return to the home that was – life will never be the same again. Although intensely painful and life-changing, however, grief is a natural reaction and entails a natural healing process. Usually it becomes less intense when we have felt and expressed our feelings of loss and anguish and, over time, have managed to make the massive integration demanded by losing a significant figure in our lives. Very gradually, we are able to adjust our thinking about ourselves and the world, and to move on to a new normality. The person who died will never be forgotten and the loss will always hurt, but he or she holds a rightful place in our memories, and life goes on.

However, although we are all programmed to recover naturally from grief, in some situations and for some of us this normal psychological process can become 'stuck'. This means that some people can experience more complicated reactions – grief that remains intense for weeks and months, or grief that is linked with upsetting images and intrusive thoughts of the deceased. An estimated 7–10 per cent of bereaved individuals (some say up to 20 per cent) experience this kind of persistent, debilitating grief, known as complicated grief (also known as unresolved, prolonged or traumatic grief). While complicated grief has been known about for many years, it was only in the 1990s that it became the focus of psychological research. Certain signs and symptoms of complicated grief were identified, mainly marked by their intensity and persistence – such as an intense yearning for the person who has died, extreme loneliness and constant preoccupation with thoughts of the dead person. It's not just that the bereaved 'can't get over it'. You may feel that life has lost its meaning, or as if part of yourself died with the person.

Complicated grief reactions have now been examined in a range of research studies that have assessed people and their psychological reactions after tragic events such as the September 11, 2001 terrorist attacks in the USA. In some studies, up to 44 per cent of people have symptoms of complicated grief. This is now accepted to the point that it was included as part of the screening that was developed as part of the public health response to people who sought support and help after the September 11 attacks.

Because grief is so individual, it can be difficult to identify complicated grief. One major clue is grief that appears to be stuck or frozen – that is, with no change at all in the grief. The grief process goes at its own pace, and may be slow and repetitive or entail more sudden change – but a particular indicator of complicated grief is the inability to move on at all, in any sense. Even after months or years, it's as if the loss has just happened. Time has stopped at the moment of bereavement; and the person remains stuck in his or her grief. Dickens describes this in *Great Expectations* in his portrait of Miss Havisham, who lives an eerie life with everything around her just as it was when her beloved 'died' to her, including a clock stopped at the moment of loss and betrayal.

People can get 'stuck' in grief for a variety of reasons – although sometimes there is no obvious cause. Factors which may make complicated grief more likely, however, include a sudden or traumatic loss, loss in early life, a prior mental or mood disorder, traumatic childhood experiences, lack of support or a close, dependent or ambivalent relationship with the deceased. Another factor can be difficulty or inability to face or process emotions.

Grief is said to become complicated when our natural psychological healing mechanisms, which exist to support recovery from distressing life events, are not effective or do not get the chance to work. In this case, 'complicated' refers to factors that interfere with the natural healing process. These factors might be related to our relationship with the person who died, our own personality and characteristics, the nature and circumstances of the death, or events that occurred after the death. Any of these, or a combination of them, may stop the natural mourning process from making us stronger and more able to cope with a world that has been changed forever.

Following bereavement, we need to find some way of regaining control and mastering the impact of the death. This book will provide you with information about the ways in which grief can become complicated, and guide you through some tried and tested ways of coping with grief.

It will outline what we know about complicated grief, both through research and through talking with people who have experienced what it is like to be 'stuck' in this way. It will explain how thoughts, feelings and behaviours can get in the way of controlling and managing the powerful impact the death of a loved one can have. There are also practical tips and exercises to help cope with the complex and overwhelming sense of loss, pain and yearning that characterizes this problem. These suggestions are based on the latest research and draw on what is known to be helpful with complicated grief. Traditional treatments for depression, such as antidepressants, may not be what's required. What appear to be most effective are therapies and exercises that help you assimilate the death on a profound level, so that you can get on with your life. These are a mixture of writing exercises and exposure therapy that gently encourage you to look at the searing emotions of grief in new ways. Sometimes talking therapies are useful too and should always be borne in mind as a possibility if required. Another focus of this book is to help you think about future goals and what you are going to do now that your loved one is gone.

The aim is to support you so that you are able to experience all the feelings linked with painful loss and to build experiences that generate more positive experiences, but in a way that does not deny or avoid the painful realities that you have had to face. In other word, try and think of this book as a safe place in which to go through such painful emotions, until you can reach a place where you can start to rebuild your life.

The exercises in this book do dig deep and may seem uncomfortable to begin with. This is because we are taking a two-pronged approach: resolving the complications and reactivating the normal mourning processes. Some research suggests that people with complicated grief have not been able to incorporate the grief at a neurological level. In one study at UCLA, assistant professor in psychoneuroimmunology Mary-Frances O'Connor and colleagues scanned the brains of women who had lost a family member following breast cancer. Most women (i.e. those with 'normal' grief) had activity in the emotional and memory centres of the brain, whereas in those with complicated grief the primary area that was activated was the nucleus accumbens, the reward centre. It was as if these women were still anticipating the reward of contact with their loved ones and had not been able to assimilate the fact that they were no longer around – even though they were perfectly aware of it consciously. Accessing such information, and incorporating new information, does take time, but can be done slowly and gently. Grief is an emotional experience that involves a very complex series of links between the thoughts that we have about ourselves as people and the way in which we relate to the world around us. Thoughts about the world after a loss tend to be specifically of our relationship with a world in which a loved one is no longer present.

1

Understanding grief and complicated grief

This chapter starts by outlining what is known about grief, and the range of ways in which people are known to respond emotionally after a death or a personally significant loss. This is followed by a more detailed outline explaining how grief reactions and psychological healing can become complicated. If you are reading this while processing your own loss and grief experience, you will be able to consider whether your own grief reaction may have been complicated by any of the factors known to interfere with natural psychological processes.

Additionally, it is easy to forget that it is not only a death or bereavement that results in loss and distress. The loss of functioning that can occur after an injury, or the loss of familiar life routines following a family breakdown, can result in intensely painful grief. Death itself is associated with a range of stressful experiences and several losses may be triggered by a death, such as loss of income or loss of access to social networks. Each of these losses can be linked with specific challenges and may make the whole process of adjustment and coping especially complex and, in some cases, complicated. Grief for a life without someone we love can be compounded if this also means a loss of important elements of life that are not provided by anyone else. Someone who loses a partner and does not have a network of supportive friends or family is more likely to struggle with grief in a way that would not occur for someone with a wide range of supportive friends. This is not to say that a large circle of friends will always be a positive factor in responding to grief – it is all very dependent on circumstances.

Grief is not something that will disappear. It will forever be associated with the loss and death experiences that have affected you so profoundly, and that you are considering as you read this book. Grief results in permanent changes in the way you feel, think and relate to other people and the world around you. This does not necessarily mean that all these changes will be negative ones; indeed, there are some changes you might make that will be very positive and may even represent improvements in certain domains of your life.

Bear in mind that, often, those who grieve profoundly are surrounded by others who are also grieving and who may be as negatively affected by the death. This can have negative effects on relationship quality, communication patterns and general satisfaction with life. In particular, studies have shown that men are usually less openly expressive of distress and less likely to confront grief and its associated emotions.

Even uncomplicated grief – i.e. grief that is not complicated by obstacles to psychological healing – has a major impact on emotional wellbeing and on all domains of life. Complicated grief results in a range of psychological symptoms that often overlap with other psychological disorders such as Post-Traumatic Stress Disorder (PTSD). Indeed, as you will see throughout the book, there are similarities between the coping techniques for grief and treatments for PTSD. Again, the intense sadness of grief overlaps with the symptoms and coping techniques helpful for Major Depressive Disorder. The remainder of this chapter will outline the ways in which grief, complicated grief, PTSD and depression are known to affect people after loss and bereavement. This will help you identify which of these psychological reactions and symptoms might be linked with your experience – a crucial first step in thinking about areas where changes could help you build your resilience and restore your psychological strength.

Acute grief

Acute grief – that is, the grief that occurs straight after a loss – is characterized by a sense of disbelief, difficulty accepting the death and an associated wide range of emotional reactions. Thoughts and memories are centred on the deceased person, and there is a narrowing in other interests. Engagement with life in general declines. Thinking is markedly focused on bereavement and related activities.

Acute grief can be thought of as a mixture of this separation response and traumatic adjustment. The following are the most common features of this:

- A sense of protest and struggle to accept the death
- An intense yearning and longing to be with the person
- A mix of other emotions, mostly painful
- A steady stream of thoughts, images, memories of the deceased
- A strong desire to reminisce and spend time with memorabilia
- Diminished interest and engagement in everyday life, mostly focused on bereavement-related activities.

Acute grief can be compared to the sort of acute inflammation that happens within the body straight after a physical injury. With this sort of sudden physical damage, the body has a healing process that gradually allows the body to return to its prior state. This may involve some pain and discomfort, but when the healing is complete, functioning returns to normal (though there may of course still be reminders of the injury, such as a scar). Sometimes the healing process is interrupted, becomes prolonged or may not happen completely. This is usually when the correct conditions for recovery are not in place – perhaps through inadequate rest or further physical strain. Try to think about grief in this way too: as something that occurs immediately after an injury that will, with the right conditions and approach to recovery and healing, resolve to become less painful. This is not the same as suggesting that 'time will heal' – it is what happens in that time that will be crucial in determining the ways in which acute grief develops immediately after a loss and bereavement.

In the vast majority of cases, this acute grief phase resolves as you acknowledge the permanent loss of the person, integrating this into your memory and mental representation. You once again become constructively occupied in daily activity, and other relationships are once again a key part of life. Although memories of the deceased can be brought to mind, these do not cause the preoccupation or prolonged and intense misery that they once did.

Understanding grief

When I trained as a clinical psychologist in the early 1990s, like many others I was introduced to the idea that there were recognizable phases through which all people pass after a bereavement. Psychiatrist Elisabeth Kübler-Ross pioneered the idea that there were stages of grieving, though these have maybe been misunderstood as being more definite than intended and were in fact first used to describe stages of acceptance in the dying, not the bereaved. Kübler-Ross's five stages – of denial, anger, bargaining, depression and acceptance – served as the foundation for much understanding about grief over many years. There is still a general expectation that reactions to bereavement proceed in a certain way over a period of time with, for example, initial shock, yearning or protest followed by despair and then restitution. Some people do still view complicated grief as characterized by a failure to pass through these stages in the prescribed order or to the predetermined timescale.

Likewise, following Freud's concept of 'grief work', Dr William Worden's four tasks of grieving form one of the best-known models of grief, whereby the process of adjustment is compared to having a series of tasks to complete:

Task 1: to accept the reality of the loss
Task 2: to experience and process the pain of grief
Task 3: to adjust to life without the person who has died
Task 4: to 'relocate' the dead person emotionally, or to find an enduring connection with him or her, and to 'move on', embarking on a new life.

For such 'grief work' to be completed, this involves going over events and memories and then working to detach from them. Such models of grief have been criticized as being too prescriptive (the 'best' way to grieve), too passive and rigid (implying that everyone should and does pass through the same tasks and stages) and too culturally specific. Research also indicates that bereaved people themselves do not feel such explanations of grief accurately reflect their experiences. In all such models, there is the notion of predetermined phases that everyone experiences, and people's grief is explained by the ways in which they fit into the sequence of tasks in the model, thus appearing to deny or bypass any individual nature of grief.

Such theories also did not seem to acknowledge that grief is a powerful emotion that often can only be handled in manageable chunks, and that grief is linked with more than the loss of the person who has died. Later clinicians such as Katherine Shear have suggested that, while there is a progression from initial disbelief and shock to painful integration of our loss, we should be much more wary of assuming that there are discrete stages and should build in more space for time away from grieving.

It is now generally accepted by psychologists that bereavement is a life event that involves stress on a number of levels, some of which can be thought of as changeable and others of which cannot. Indeed, within psychology generally it is also recognized much more nowadays that the differences between so-called 'normal' psychological reactions and reactions classified as 'unhealthy' or 'unhelpful' are more likely to be related to how often thoughts, feelings or behaviours occur and how intensely this happens. More is now known about effective and ineffective coping strategies, and in many ways it makes much more sense to ask whether coping strategies are effective for individuals, rather than to classify patterns of coping as being more or less a sign of good or bad adjustment.

Many models of coping examine the way in which people classify stressful problems, either as 'problems to be solved and fixed' or 'emotions that need to be handled because they cannot be fixed'. Some have proposed that 'problem-focused coping' is associated with better health and wellbeing and 'emotion-focused coping' is not. If only understanding coping and adjustment were that simple! Emotion-focused coping may be helpful or unhelpful. This book will help you to think about your coping responses, how to understand these and how to make any changes that might be helpful in adjusting to changes after a death or other significant loss.

A 'common wisdom' seems to have become established in society and within the helping professions generally that it is healthy to focus on the pain and distress and to express it openly. Doing so was considered 'normal' in the days and weeks after a death, while suppressing or 'keeping a lid on' the grief and distressing emotions was thought to be 'unhealthy' and not to be encouraged. This advice is still commonly given and is very much based on the notion that confronting the pain of loss is an essential element of 'coming to terms' with it, and necessary if subsequent physical and mental health problems are to be avoided. However, researchers have examined many elements of this received wisdom and have shown that it is not supported by evidence. In particular, this wisdom doesn't acknowledge how exhausting continuing confrontation can be for the grieving person.

Margaret Stroebe, professor of bereavement and loss at Utrecht University, recognized that it is not as simple as confronting a loss. Nor does non-confrontation automatically mean mal-adaptation. In addition to the need to face grief, pain and distress, there is also a natural urge to avoid the reality of the death and its consequences – and this should be factored in, as it is beneficial. Avoidance can have a valuable protective effect for the person struggling to make sense of an overwhelming loss.

The dual process model of coping with bereavement

In recent years, there has been a significant amount of research into what is known as the 'dual process' model of grief (DPM) by clinicians such as Margaret Stroebe and Katherine Shear. The dual process posits a more dynamic and complex process of coping with grief than submitting to stages. Roughly, it is based on oscillation, whereby the bereaved confronts his or her loss at times and avoids it at other times. The person 'swings' between facing his or her loss and restoration, or rebuilding his or her life. 'Time out' is an essential feature of this, based on the knowledge that grief is 'arduous and exhausting', as Margaret Stroebe says. In other words, the DPM allows room for the benefits of avoidance at times. People cannot always be looking the pain of grief in the face, and need time off if they are to recover and function. The DPM also takes into account the fact that other sources of life stress may exist in addition to the death itself, such as financial worries or being left alone to bring up children.

Mourning, then, is viewed as an instinctive activity, where the loss is processed – but not all at once. Adjustment to our loss proceeds in 'fits and starts', as Katherine Shear puts it. Coming to terms with a death is characterized by moving attention towards detail of the painful loss and, paradoxically, away from it. This moving away from the pain of the loss has sometimes been referred to as 'defensive exclusion', in which we need time off from reality. We need a balance between paying attention to the loss and to the issues that need to be confronted in order to restore our previous interest and engagement in life functioning.

As Shear says,

> Adjustment occurs during a period of acute grief, during which confrontation with the painful reality oscillates with defensive exclusion, in the form of numbing, focus on positive memories, imagined reunion, and other forms of respite in which attention is directed toward neutral or positive thoughts.

(Shear 2010)

So in the early stages after a death it is normal for you to alternate between periods of intense distress and defensive exclusion. You may discover that you have periods where your thoughts are more about positive memories of the person who has died. This is encouraging and a sign that your mind is acknowledging that, in the longer term, it will be more helpful for you to have a set of memories that encompass all the person's life, not only the more recent and more accessible recollections around the time of his or her death – that is, the ones that have been so dominant and difficult to cope with.

Terms such as 'positive growth', 'reconstruction of meaning' and 'creating a narrative' have also been used to describe ways in which grief and bereavement should be linked with a return to a positive state of mind and wellbeing as soon as possible.

The DPM model has been developed by Professors Stroebe and Schut and has been reproduced as Figure 1.1 (overleaf) with their kind permission.

As you can see, in the DPM the pendulum of the griever swings between loss-oriented strategies and restoration-oriented strategies. This is the main difference between the DPM and other models of grief. Loss-oriented strategies refer to times when thinking, behaviour and feelings are focused on loss. Restoration-oriented strategies

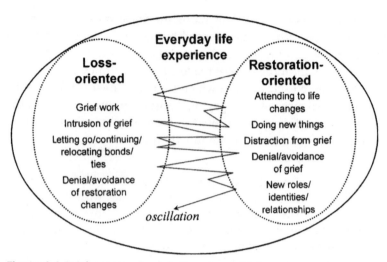

Figure 1.1 Dual process model of coping with bereavement
(Stroebe and Schut 1999: p. 13, reproduced by permission)

are when thinking, behaviour and feelings are focused on restoring elements of life that help with coping with grief. It's important to bear these opposite strategies in mind as you read this book, because typically the person with complicated grief will be much more loss-oriented – that is, much more focused on loss.

Resolution and moving forward are themes common to many of the models of understanding grief. A key need is to accept the reality of the loss and the reality of the wider changed world following a death. But, as the DPM notes, adjusting to life after a death involves having to master all the changes in one's personal and wider environment, as well as 'relocating' the dead person emotionally and 'moving on'. The dual process model acknowledges that there is a need to develop new roles, identities and relationships, although grief proceeds at its own pace.

Integrated grief

It is important to explain what 'integrated grief' means and how this relates to complicated grief. The goal of integrating all the complex facets of grief into one experience where loss-related memories can be brought to mind without being intensely overwhelming is at the heart of the move from complicated to integrated grief.

Complicated grief is more likely to happen when this integration cannot be achieved. With integrated grief, feelings of grief occur from time to time and, unlike acute grief, there is a comprehension of the death and how it is understood and experienced in relation to wider thoughts of self and the world.

Thoughts and memories of the deceased person can be accessed in consciousness, but this does not result in preoccupation or the characteristic pattern of 'yo-yoing' between overwhelming emotion and strong desires to avoid and push the impact on emotion and thoughts out of the mind. Engagement in all domains of life is re-established when grief is integrated, and quality of life rises, in contrast with acute grief where there is partial, limited or no engagement with important life domains.

Complicated grief is characterized by prolonged suffering and an inability to find avenues for meaningful and personally fulfilling activities – more time is focused on loss than on restoration. Coping with important life problems that are triggered by the grief can also cause complications. Sometimes the bereavement itself is described as being complicated, referring to difficult and challenging circumstances of the death, problematic relationships with the deceased person or difficult or challenging consequences of the death. However, if there is a complicated set of circumstances leading to a death or complex relationships that influence the reactions to a death, this does not automatically mean that a grief reaction will be complicated.

Grief by itself does not constitute depression, nor is it a mental disorder. However, it can sometimes trigger the development of other psychological symptoms, such as Post-Traumatic Stress Disorder or major depression. Like these, complicated grief can impair day-to-day functioning and there is overlap – such as low self-worth and thoughts of suicide in depression, or intrusive thoughts of the deceased, avoidance of reminders and emotional numbness in PTSD.

Some clinicians and researchers have noted that people report symptoms of PTSD and major depression along with complicated grief, thus prompting the question of whether they are the same thing. This continues to be a matter of debate, along with whether it is possible or even necessary to understand the links between them. They are usually viewed as separate entities, although treatment may be very similar – interestingly, treatment for complicated grief originally grew out of treatment for PTSD.

Post-Traumatic Stress Disorder

PTSD is an anxiety disorder characterized by the person re-experiencing a trauma through unwanted and intrusive images or memories of a traumatic event, avoidance of situations related to the trauma and physical symptoms such as being startled and jumpy at reminders of the traumatic event.

Approximately 20–30 per cent of people develop symptoms of PTSD after bereavement, often referred to as 'clusters' of symptoms. These clusters are known as 're-experiencing', 'avoidance' and 'arousal' symptom clusters:

- *Re-experiencing symptoms*: details of the bereavement are repeatedly relived. These are most commonly experienced as flashbacks, nightmares or intrusive memories, making the person feel as though the entire event is happening all over again. It's the intrusive quality which is characteristic (grabbing the attention), along with the feeling of the event being replayed.
- *Avoidance* is characterized by efforts to avoid reminders of the deceased person and triggers related to the death, whether that's in terms of situations, feelings or thoughts.
- *Arousal symptoms* are generally related to a range of emotional reactions in response to the other symptom clusters. They usually relate to anxiety (including exaggerated startle responses), disturbed sleep or feeling emotionally numb in relation to the trauma.

Although there is of course a 'traumatic element' to the experiences that happen when grieving, not everyone who has intense grief will experience PTSD or these symptoms, although some people with complicated grief may have some symptoms of PTSD. A feature of complicated grief is the unwanted thoughts and reminders of loss and death that cause intense distress and changes in behaviour. In complicated grief there is an intense desire to think about the person who has died; people have a desire to be near to reminders, unlike in PTSD where there is an urge to avoid reminders, stay away and keep the reminders at bay. If you have concerns that you have any of these symptoms, speak with your GP or a healthcare professional who will be able to advise you.

Major Depressive Disorder

More serious symptoms of depression can develop, where depressed and sad moods predominate and do not change from day to day. People with major depressive symptoms do not experience pleasure from activities that they previously enjoyed and tend to think of themselves critically. Sleep and appetite become disturbed, energy and motivation are significantly diminished and people may feel intensely irritable and guilty. The feeling that life is not worth living and sometimes thoughts of suicide can occur, as can feelings of hopelessness and pessimism.

Seeking professional help

Elements of post-traumatic symptoms and depression are of course often experienced as a 'normal' consequence of grief and loss, and the occurrence of these symptoms does not necessarily mean that a diagnosis of PTSD or depression is warranted or that there is necessarily a need for specialist therapy or treatment. As already mentioned and as we will explain in later chapters, management often involves similar techniques and strategies.

Much research has been carried out into understanding the psychological responses to life events and the way in which psychological problems may manifest. However, health and social care professionals often do not understand psychological reactions to bereavement in similar or consistent ways. For example, the initial reaction to a death as described on page 2, 'acute grief', can present itself to clinical staff in a variety of ways, depending on the nature of the bereavement and the person experiencing the loss. Because of the variation in understanding, acute grief reactions can sometimes be wrongly labelled by professionals as 'pathological' or 'complicated'. This can be distressing and damaging, and may lead to unhelpful ways of thinking.

Many GPs and some mental health professionals might not necessarily be able to distinguish the differences between acute grief reactions, PTSD, major depression and/or complicated grief reactions. Fortunately, in terms of treatment this usually isn't crucial, as there is sufficient overlap in psychological and pharmacological therapies to mean that people in distress should be able to access help and support. In more complex cases, or when supportive care interventions are not helping, this lack of professional understanding may become more crucial.

If you are in contact with your GP or healthcare professional, you should advise them that you are planning to undertake some self-help work to cope with complications arising from your grief. The key information that they will want to know is outlined on page x so that you can provide this to them.

This book is based on work that recognizes a specific cluster of symptoms referred to as complicated grief. It has been demonstrated that this requires a specific approach to support resolution, based on helping people to confront painful emotions about grief that are initially avoided and on supporting them in gaining control over avoidance and exposure to thinking about death and how this can be incorporated into their beliefs to promote adjustment for the future. The exercises in this book aim to encourage a two-pronged approach to coping with grief, removing the obstacles so natural psychological healing can take place. If you are in contact with a healthcare professional who is prescribing medication, or with a counsellor or psychological therapist, it is important for them to continue to co-ordinate your care and treatment.

Questions for reflection and self-awareness

Throughout this book you will be encouraged to think about and write down your responses to exercises on coping with reactions and adjustment to grief. There is a vocabulary around grief. You may hear people around you using such terms and you may not have thought about how language contributes to your own awareness and thoughts about what you have been experiencing.

Throughout this book I will outline some questions designed to help you consider the content of each chapter and how it might apply to your experiences. I will include questions that might help you think about how you and those important to you have understood complicated grief. You will find it helpful to have a notebook for your responses.

Exercise 1.1

Having considered an initial introduction to grief and grief reactions, what words used do you particularly identify with? 'Acute', 'prolonged', 'complicated', 'integrated'? Write these in your notebook.

Exercise 1.2

Think about the following, and write your responses in your notebook:

- In which ways did your acute grief show itself?
- What have you avoided doing since your loss?
- What do you tend to avoid thinking about now, since your bereavement?
- What are some of the things that you think about grief?
- Have you ever sat down to consider grief and what it means to you?
- Have you observed events or had experiences within your personal life or within the world in general that have influenced your understanding and experience of grief?

2

Understanding your grief reactions

The previous chapter outlined ways in which acute grief occurs after a death or bereavement, showing how for some people this becomes complicated. Loss-related thinking and emotions start to dominate life, and there are difficulties integrating this with other elements of life, restoring normality or linking the experience in a meaningful way with thoughts about the world. In other words, your world perspective becomes skewed by grief, and this stance can take on a life of its own and become hard to break.

Acute grief is characterized by disbelief, and difficulty comprehending the final nature of the death and its associated losses. There is intense sadness and longing that usually oscillates in intensity. There are recurrent and distracting thoughts of the dead person and a lack of interest in things that are unrelated to the deceased, resulting in an unsettling feeling of incompetence. Complicated grief is different. This chapter outlines the features of complicated grief, gives some theories on its source, and will help you think about whether this is what has happened to you and, if so, how it may affect your day-to-day life.

Beginning to understand your responses to complicated grief can be the first step in making sense of what has happened and beginning to recover.

What is complicated grief?

Complicated grief is when acute grief symptoms remain overly intense and do not change over time. Strong feelings of longing for the person who has died can interfere with thinking or feeling anything else, hampering your ability to return to a normal routine and to access other areas in order to build and restore quality of life. Such grief is more likely when certain aspects of the death are too painful to think about. There may be inability to accept or process the circumstances of someone's death, leading to continuing pain and complicated grief. A typical thought is that 'if only' something different had happened, the person would not have died – if the medical staff had been quicker or more helpful, say, or if the bereaved person had acted with more thought or speed.

A feature of complicated grief is intense preoccupation with the dead person, to the point where you are unable to think about anything else. To a certain extent this happens in all grief, of course, and preoccupation is part of any normal grief reaction – it is the dominance of the reaction that makes this a characteristic element of complex grief.

Paul was widowed at 45 when his wife died of cancer, leaving him with three teenage children. He was quite unable to cope, and shut himself off from the world. He had no close friends and his wife had been everything to him. He refused to engage with his children and had progressively less to do with them as time went on, retreating more and more into a world of his own. Indeed, his children felt that he blamed them for the death, as being too demanding of their mother's time and attention. When he died 30 years later, it was found that he had kept everything belonging to his wife, right down to the last yellowed old nightie.

Rob's father killed himself in Rob's bedroom when Rob was 14. Rob, now 21, is unable to have a conversation without bringing this in after a few minutes. He is in desperate need of therapy but seems unable to make the least start in understanding his grief, or even to move beyond the point of trauma when his father shot himself.

Maria is a young widow whose husband died suddenly of a heart attack just four days after the birth of her second child. Eleven years on, it's as if the death has only just happened, and she still speaks of it all as if she had only lost her husband the other day, going over the demise and funeral in obsessive detail. She has had two lots of therapy and is now embarking on a third with clinicians specializing in traumatic loss.

Chrissie lost her father at age 94. Although his demise was more than expected, she was stunned by the reality of the death, and irrationally felt that she could and should have done more to prevent it. Her life remained on hold for two years, during which she suffered acute guilt and depression. She believed this was compounded by her difficult relationship with her father and the sheer exhaustion of having looked after him for a number of years beforehand. Cognitive Behavioural Therapy (CBT) and antidepressants (which we'll discuss in Chapter 5) very gradually helped, and after two years Chrissie made a full recovery even though, as she says, to a life that is new and different and sometimes a little scary.

Susan lost her husband of 30 years and was devastated. She kept hearing his voice and seeing him everywhere, and would scan the street for glimpses of him. So haunted was she by his presence, it was impossible for her to re-engage in everyday life. Her family were shocked and concerned, as Susan had always been a vibrant, energetic, involved person. But now she was obsessed by the feeling that 'if only I had done more' she could have prevented his death. Eventually, with her family's persuasion, she sought help and benefited from some of the techniques in this book. In particular, she found it very helpful to make a detailed record of the circumstances of her husband's death (see Chapter 3) and to have an imaginary conversation with him, in which she was able to voice all the feelings and concerns she'd been holding in, unable to share with anyone else (see Chapter 7).

Common features of complicated grief

- It is long-lasting: if symptoms last for at least six months it is not likely that they will improve without intervention, and it is this sort of reaction that has been studied most often in relation to complicated grief.
- It is intrusive (or attention-grabbing), with repeated images and mental pictures related to the death and/or its consequences.
- Preoccupation is another feature – when a person is not able to stop thinking about something. There are strong memories of the person who has died, and at the same time there may be a tendency to push away the pain as much as possible and to take steps to avoid thinking about the person who has died. Paul, for example, was unable to look at his wife's clothes and left them hanging in the cupboard until he himself passed on.
- Quality of life is also profoundly affected – again, this is normal during grief but lasts much longer in complicated grief. People with complicated grief are less likely to have contact with others, and will have fewer outings. They may take less exercise, and eating and sleeping habits may change, usually for the worse.

There is much debate as to whether complicated grief should be classed as a mental disorder, and indeed whether it is right or appropriate to pathologize it in this way. At the time of writing, the precise diagnostic criteria for complicated grief are under debate, but commonly agreed characteristics include:

- Yearning, pining or longing for the deceased
- Trouble accepting the death
- Feeling uneasy about moving on with one's life
- Inability to trust others since the death
- Excessive bitterness or anger about the death
- Persistent feeling of being shocked, stunned or emotionally numb since the death
- Frequent intense feelings of loneliness
- Feeling that life is empty or meaningless without the deceased (refraining from doing things or going to places that remind one of the loss)
- Frequent preoccupying thoughts about the person who died.

The *British Medical Journal* has described complicated grief as 'the persistent and disruptive yearning, pining and longing for the deceased'. It has stated the following as being symptomatic of complicated grief:

- Frequent trouble accepting the death
- Inability to trust others since the death
- Excessive bitterness related to the death
- Uneasiness about moving on with life
- Detachment from other people to whom the bereaved person was previously close
- The prolonged feeling that life is meaningless
- The view that the future will never hold any prospect of fulfilment
- Excessive and prolonged agitation since the death.

Some people might think that surely grief is always complicated. Complex, yes. There are often all sorts of emotions to be processed – huge sadness, regret and the ramifications of fraught relationships. But, as I've said, sooner or later grief usually runs its course. The loss is not forgotten, but assimilated. You have come to terms with it, however painful and prolonged the process. But with complicated grief you are, as it were, living in an eternal present of grief, stuck in the pain. There is no movement. Complicated grief gets a grip – a stranglehold, even – on life and it is impossible to 'make peace' or reach a sense of resolution following the death. You might feel that time is moving on and you are not. You or others may have noted that the mourning process seems to be stuck, derailed or unresolved.

Maybe there is something about the death that keeps coming back to your mind, a sense that things will never make sense and no sign that this is lessening as the weeks and months pass you by. You may even find that you cannot actually concentrate on the loss itself, as there is something you cannot get out of your mind – something that keeps coming back to you, grabbing your attention and generating strong feelings of distress and a longing to turn back the clock. You may have been coping by excessive drinking, over-eating or seeking refuge in other behaviours that have a detrimental impact on your mental and physical wellbeing.

Your life may feel empty, and the loneliness is difficult to cope with. You may become isolated from people, perhaps because some friends were contacts of the person who has died. In addition, even when you are physically in contact with other people, it is common to feel disconnected from them emotionally. This can be a protective measure. When you are in the grip of strong emotions relating to loss and separation, the last thing you feel up to is risking more potential loss by investing time and attention in a relationship that might not work out. Although people will be considerate and probably won't ask much of you, some may well encourage you to move back into the world. If friends and family are telling you that you need to move on, then this could be a clue that you are experiencing some of the signs of complicated grief.

Intrusive images and memories

Many people with complicated grief are haunted by upsetting memories. Every time you fall asleep you may experience distressing imagery or memories of the person who has died. If so, take heart. These can be a doorway into healing. Part of understanding your grief is to make sense of the very images, memories and the linked feelings that you experience. Over a few days, pay attention to and note down the images or memories that come into your mind most often. These could be small fragments of memories or images as opposed to a fully formed sequence of events and information. This is all right, so don't be too concerned if this is the case: just aim to gather the information at this point. Trying to make sense of what it means or how it relates to coping with grief can be managed later.

Exercise 2.1 is an example of an image log. In your notebook, create your own image log to note any imagery that occurs when you are experiencing feelings of grief. This may be an image that has a beginning, middle and end, like a video clip, or it could just be parts of images and mental pictures that come to mind. At this point do not be too concerned about which sort of image you experience: all that is important at this point is for you to record it in your notebook.

Exercise 2.1

Date and time	Image details
Monday 11 p.m.	Picture of him lying in bed, looking so grey and when he could hardly lift his head from the pillow

There are emotions that occur following death that can be thought of as natural and almost universal. It is important to be able to recognize these, understand their origins and be aware of how best to respond and react.

- Which emotions have you noticed most often following your bereavement?
- What did you learn as a child about emotions and expressing them?
- Do you truly feel, experience and express these? If not, why not?
- What would need to happen for you to feel able to express these emotions?
- When you express the feeling, does this lead to any changes in your experience of emotions?
- If not, might it be that you are holding back in some way or not fully stating how you feel emotionally?

- Are there any factors that might have interfered with your normal recovery from grief?

You may find it helpful to record your answers in your notebook.

As you know, grief is not the only emotion that you will be experiencing. When you are grieving, you experience a wide range of feelings in addition to sadness. Think about some of these other strong emotions you have experienced along with or in response to grief and write them down in your notebook.

Thoughts about grief and emotional reactions can also significantly influence behavioural reactions and coping strategies. Beliefs that 'grief will overwhelm me' can lead to numbing and a wide range of avoidance tactics. These beliefs often link back to significant experiences earlier in life, possibly though not always relating to childhood. However, have a think about this, and again, here are some questions to help you:

- What did you learn about grief and emotion as a child?
- What do you think other people's reactions would be now if you expressed emotion?
- Do you have any strong or significant memories of someone else expressing grief or a strong emotion?
- If so, what happened? How did other people react?
- Can you think about what you might have learned or what sense you might have made of this at the time?

Avoidance of the consequences of grief and expression of the emotional consequences of grief can become a fixed and inflexible coping response, especially as the benefits of avoidance are very powerful reinforcers – avoidance is helpful in the short term and this means it is more likely to keep on happening because of the positive benefits. Avoidance also interferes with the processing of information that is needed to make sense of the grief and to re-order beliefs and priorities in life. However, avoidance can also be helpful and support adaption to life after a death and coping with the impact. These helpful periods of avoidance can be thought of as periods of respite.

Understanding the impact of complicated grief

Take some time to think about your levels of grief, yearning or longing, and use this as a way of understanding your current feelings, thoughts and reactions to the pain of your loss. Try to think of these signs as your body and mind's way of reminding you that there has been a significant assault on you (remember the example in Chapter 1 about how the body reacts to an acute physical injury) and that you need to discover how best to recover and build the strength needed to promote natural psychological healing.

- Notice when and how much you have any times of strong grief, yearning or longing – make some notes on what sorts of situations trigger this. This will help you notice the ways in which complicated grief is manifesting in your own life.
- What are the predominant memories and thoughts you have been noticing about the person who died? It may be that because of the pain of your grief you cannot face thinking about memories, though taking it slowly and in a gradual and controlled way might be helpful.

If you notice that your levels of enjoyment and interest are not changing then you should think about speaking with a healthcare professional about whether you may have symptoms of a clinically significant depressive reaction.

How might thoughts and beliefs about grief affect your reactions?

As we saw in Chapter 1, many healthcare professionals, and many people in general, subscribe to the theory that there are stages of grief and grieving, believing that there are a discrete number and sequence of phases through which grieving people should pass. These often encapsulate myths of grief and mourning, which could inform the sort of advice that other people have given you. You might need to think about how you will respond if people (including healthcare professionals) provide you with advice that is at odds with what this book recommends for addressing the complications that have occurred with your grief reactions.

If you notice that you are having extreme and powerful reactions to other people's comments about recovery, elements of your experience that suggest your grief might be less intense or advice on how to cope in general, then this may be a 'warning sign' that the comment has touched on an area where you are still trying to make sense of how your prior beliefs and thoughts can fit with life after the loss and change in your life.

Consider the following list of symptoms to help you think about whether you have been experiencing any features of complicated grief. These are taken from the criteria developed by a group of clinicians who think that complicated grief should be regarded as a separate disorder in its own right. There are common systems of classification for psychological or mental health problems, the most commonly used being the *Diagnostic and Statistical Manual of Mental Disorders* (*DSM*) and also the fifth chapter of the *International Classification of Diseases*. Complicated grief does not appear specifically in these, though researchers in this area have developed criteria to illustrate how this would be considered if further research confirmed the benefit of inclusion.

Classification of complicated grief

You experienced the death of a close family member or close friend at least 12 months ago. In the case of bereaved children, the death may have occurred at least six months ago. At least one of the following symptoms of persistent intense acute grief has been present for a period longer than is expected by others in the person's social or cultural environment:

- Persistent intense yearning or longing for the person who died (in young children, yearning may be expressed in play and behaviour, including separation–reunion behaviour with caregivers)
- Frequent intense feelings of loneliness; feeling that life is empty or meaningless without the person who died
- Recurrent thoughts that it is unfair, meaningless or unbearable to have to live when a loved one has died, or a recurrent urge to die in order to find or join the deceased
- Frequent preoccupying thoughts about the person who died, e.g.

thoughts or images of the person intrude on usual activities or interfere with functioning.

There may be preoccupation with the circumstances of the death. In children, this may be expressed through play and behaviour, and may extend to preoccupation with the possible death of others close to them.

At least two of the following symptoms are present for at least a month:

- Frequent troubling rumination about the circumstances of the death or its consequences, e.g. concerns about how or why the person died, about not being able to manage without the loved one, of having let the deceased person down, etc.
- Recurrent feeling of disbelief or inability to accept the death; the person cannot believe or accept that the loved one is really gone
- Persistent feeling of being shocked, stunned, dazed or emotionally numb since the death
- Recurrent feelings of anger or bitterness related to the death.

Some people may also have difficulty with any positive reminiscing about the person who has died. For example, they may tend to indulge in excessive self-blame and avoidance of any reminder of the loss and death, avoiding people, situations or places associated with the person.

There is also usually a disruption in social function and self-identity. This is shown through:

- A desire to die in order to be with the deceased
- Difficulty trusting other individuals since the death
- Feeling alone or detached from other individuals since the death
- Feeling that life is meaningless or empty without the deceased or the belief that one cannot function without the deceased
- Confusion about one's role in life or a diminished sense of one's identity (e.g. feeling that a part of oneself died with the deceased)
- Difficulty or reluctance to pursue interests since the loss or to plan for the future (e.g. friendships, activities).

The bereavement reaction must be out of proportion or inconsistent with cultural, religious or age-appropriate norms. Following a death that occurred under traumatic circumstances (e.g. homicide, suicide, disaster or accident), there could be persistent, frequent and distressing thoughts, images or feelings related to traumatic features of the death (e.g. the deceased's degree of suffering, gruesome injury, blame of self or others for the death), including in response to reminders of the loss. In the proposed diagnostic systems this would be recognized as Complicated Grief following a Traumatic Bereavement.

Your reactions

Do you get images or memories of the person who died which you would describe as 'intrusive' – that is, unwanted in the way that they grab your attention when you would rather be thinking of something else? It is thought that these ruminations, or preoccupation with thoughts of the deceased person, make it more difficult to come to terms with the reality of the loss and its distress. Although you are thinking about the person (which means that the reality and pain are not being avoided), the rumination or repetitive quality of the thinking means that you don't gain any new insights into how best to respond, or how to work out the way in which your beliefs could be causing problems with overall adjustment and psychological healing.

You may have experienced thoughts that it is not 'right' or appropriate that you experience positive emotions or enjoyment from activities. These thoughts often have their origins in myths that there is a specific period of time when you should be mourning – and a time when this should have stopped or be less intense. You might be concerned about the thoughts of others if they were to see you engaged in certain activities that they think you 'should not' be involved with so soon (or at all) after a death. This sort of concern is illustrative of the rigidity of expectation about grief and grieving – not acknowledging that this is always a very individual decision and something that cannot be prescribed or predefined. Anger about the actions of other people or at 'the world' in general is common. If you have been feeling angry, try to work out with whom and with what.

Here are some more questions to help you with gaining awareness of your reactions. Remember, it is absolutely not the case that there is a predictable sequence or a defined series of steps through which someone must pass in order to be regarded as grieving normally.

- Are you able to visit the final resting place of the deceased person?
- Have you been able to engage in thinking about or doing the things that you used to do with the deceased person?
- Have you been able to visit the places that you used to visit together?
- What are the common day-to-day reminders that intensify your feelings of loss?
- How do you react when this happens?

Has your grief reaction become complicated?

Several questionnaires have been developed to assess the symptoms and features of complicated grief. An example is reproduced on page 26 to help you further think about the extent to which these are features of your response, and to help you decide which self-help approaches are best for you. This can also help you to measure changes over time, and to structure a conversation with any healthcare professionals who might be involved in supporting you in adjusting to a death.

Various questions may help determine whether grief has become complicated. Consider each of those listed below and write down your responses in your notebook:

- Are you having trouble accepting the death?
- Does grief interfere with your life?
- Are you having troublesome or preoccupying images or thoughts of the person who has died?
- Are there things that you used to do when your loved one was alive that you don't feel comfortable doing any more, or that you avoid?
- Are you feeling cut off or distant from other people since the death?

Exercise 2.2

Consider the following questions (from the Traumatic Grief Inventory) and provide a score of 0 for never, 1 for rarely, 2 for sometimes, 3 for often and 4 for always.

1 I think about this person so much that it's hard for me to do the things I normally do.
2 Memories of the person who died upset me.
3 I cannot accept the death of the person who died.
4 I feel myself longing for the person who died.
5 I feel drawn to places and things associated with the person who died.
6 I can't help feeling angry about my loved one's death.
7 I feel disbelief over what happened.
8 I feel stunned or dazed about what happened.
9 Ever since my loved one died it has been hard for me to trust people.
10 Ever since my loved one died I feel I have lost the ability to care about other people, or I feel distant from people I care about.
11 I have pain in the same area of my body or I have some of the same symptoms as the person who died.
12 I go out of my way to avoid reminders of the person who died.
13 I feel that life is empty without the person who died.
14 I hear the voice of the person who died speaking to me.
15 I see the person who died standing before me.
16 I feel that it is unfair that I should live when this person died.
17 I feel bitter over this person's death.
18 I feel envious of others who have not lost someone close.
19 I feel lonely a great deal of the time ever since my loved one died.

When you have added up your score, note it down. If your total score is greater than 24 you should discuss this with a healthcare professional, with a view to seeking professional support.

Consider the following list and note down those that have applied to you in the past month.

- Have you felt yourself longing and yearning for your loved one every day?
- Has the yearning been distressing to you or disruptive to your daily routine?

How many of the following apply to you?

- You have had difficulty accepting the death.

- You have had difficulty trusting people.
- You have felt bitter about the death.
- You have felt uneasy about moving on in your life.
- You have felt a sense of numbness or had difficulty connecting with other people.
- You have felt that life was empty or meaningless without the lost person.
- You have felt that the future holds no meaning or purpose without him or her.
- You have felt on edge, jumpy or easily startled.

If more than half of the above apply to you, you could have a complicated grief reaction.

Grief as the status quo

Although it may seem difficult to take on board, people may actually find it preferable and easier to focus on their distress and grief rather than to begin to think about how to engage with their lives. They may have no way of conceiving of how their daily lives might now be experienced in the aftermath of a death. Grief can become a state of being that serves a positive function in and of itself – that is, it becomes a status quo, which though not exactly comfortable is at least familiar. Moreover, although painful and challenging, grief can be the only link left with the person and, as such, there is an understandable reluctance to 'give this up'. Sometimes, too, people become concerned about what others will think of them if they are no longer seen to be grieving. What else could you do to retain a deep sense of connection with the person who has died? If you are not sure about this at the moment then come back to this question when you have considered some of the other content in the remainder of the book.

Myths of mourning

Dr Therese Rando has described the 'myths of mourning' as outlined below:

- Grief and the amount of time spent mourning or focusing on the death decline steadily after the death.

- All deaths and losses prompt the same type of grief and mourning reactions.
- Following a bereavement, people need only express their feelings in order to resolve their mourning.
- In order to be healthier and have a greater sense of adjustment it is necessary for people to put thoughts of the dead person out of their mind.
- Grief is predominantly a reaction that impacts on people psychologically and mentally.
- The intensity of emotions related to grief and the amount of time for which a grief reaction is experienced is a testimony to how much love there was for the deceased.
- Grief and loss are only about the loss of the person and nothing else.
- Death is the same no matter what happened before it – sudden and unexpected deaths are essentially the same as deaths that are anticipated.
- Time heals all psychological pain and grief gets better on its own with time.

Having read some of these myths, are there any that you identify with or feel are ones you or those close to you have believed? These are all myths that do not fit with the findings of psychological research into grief and grieving. For example, the amount of time that elapses after a loss does not necessarily result in a lessening in the intensity of grief or the amount of thinking time devoted to the death and its impact. Although some general principles have been highlighted through research, each individual set of reactions will be uniquely determined by the individual relationships involved. Again, research also suggests that tactics such as expressing feelings or pushing thoughts away are not likely to be helpful long-term solutions *per se*.

When thinking and beliefs get in the way of healing

People tend to have a natural tendency to resist information that is at odds with their existing mindsets. There is an understandable reaction against the need for changes in thinking and beliefs after a death, particularly when it was not expected or anticipated, or when elements of the experience were not a part of an existing mindset. Acknowledging the permanence of the death and having to readjust and reconstruct previously held thoughts and beliefs about the person who has died (as well as about life) is tremendously difficult. However, it is often only when this has happened that readjustment of life goals and expectations can occur.

When someone close to us dies, beliefs about trust, safety, fairness and control in relation to life, living and the world in general can be shattered. For instance, if someone believed that the world was a fair place to live in and then experienced the sudden death of a child in a road accident, it would be difficult for that person to hold on to the belief that the world was a fair place when something so tragic and seemingly unfair could happen.

There are two ways in which mental responses to loss and grief can be developed. First, information is altered so that prior beliefs about self and the world are not changed. The person whose child has been tragically killed may start to believe that the event is in some way related to punishment for a prior event. This allows her to 'keep' her belief that the world is a fair place, explaining the seemingly unjust and unfair accident as an isolated occurrence related to perceived punishment. There will be positive consequences for her in that this does not require her to embark upon the work of 'revising' her belief system, though there is a downside in relation to the depression and shame that will be linked with the belief that she is being punished. This mental response pattern is called assimilation.

To check whether this is your response pattern, consider the following questions:

- Have you been able to fit your death experience with what you already believed about the world?
- Did you think that what has happened to you has happened to other people?
- What did you think about this before the death?
- Is there anything that has happened since the death that has been a personal shock or revelation with regard to your previous way of seeing things?

The second way that reactions can occur is when prior beliefs are changed to incorporate new information that is encountered as a result of the loss and grief. If the mother above had reacted in this way instead of viewing the accident as self-punishment, she might have considered it as exceedingly painful and not something that she ever thought would happen to her, but at the same time would be able to recognize that there are some elements of life that are 'just', predictable and controllable. This reaction is known as accommodation.

Assimilation and accommodation are technical terms used to explain how the beliefs and thoughts you held before the death change in line with differences in your thinking afterwards. Both processes are about making sense of what has happened. The first is when you explain the death to yourself according to what you have always believed about the world; the second is when you don't have a way of easily explaining it and therefore have to come up with explanations or thoughts that help to do so. When beliefs are altered in more extreme ways, this often serves to help people feel safer and more in control. Here are some examples of thoughts that some people experience when accommodating the impact of grief and loss into their belief systems:

- I can never love again.
- This is so painful that I can't experience positive emotions again in the future.

This change in belief, although associated with depression, keeps the person safe from experiencing the hurt and pain of loving someone who has died.

Attachment and separation responses

As human beings, we are instinctively pre-programmed to seek, establish and maintain close relationships with other people. Separation and the loss of these relationships results in recognized responses. This instinctive pull towards close relationships has been called the 'bio-behavioural attachment system' and operates throughout life. Wellbeing and good psychological functioning are achieved when there is a strong and secure sense of attachment. It is thought that we tend to have up to five attachment relationships at any one time in our lives.

There are sections in our memory that store details about our attachment and caregiving relationships. These contain information that is within our awareness (called explicit memory) as well as information that is out of our awareness. Such memories tend to guide our predictions about life and influence our behavioural reactions, including the way in which we respond to problems that are specific to a relationship.

Effectively, this is a special form of longer-term memory which helps organize and order our feelings, as well as informing expectations of our own and others' reactions in relationships. Research has shown that these specific memory stores hold information about each significant attachment relationship that we have; this is sometimes referred to as the working 'mental model' of the relationship. Indeed, this working model may be what makes it possible for us to be separated from key people in our lives – in our minds we have a clear 'working model' of how the relationship operates that we can access when they are not present.

So, this mental model – of the person as a vital source of comfort, love and caregiving – is initially very resistant to processing the new information that the person has died. This strong separation response can trigger the common feeling after a death that the lost person might reappear ('I can't believe he's not just going to walk through the door at any moment'), along with yearning and longing to be with the person. As Shear has noted, 'People do not forget loved ones who die, nor do they stop caring for them. Instead they feel a permanent sense of connection and responsibility to the person who died' (Shear 2010).

Many of the symptoms that are part of complicated grief are the result of this separation. They continue to be experienced despite the passage of time: the separation does not become any less painful, as it is not possible to lessen the pain through contact or time spent with the person (as might be the case when the pain of separation happens for other reasons, such as travel away or temporary separation for other reasons).

This reaction can be understood by thinking about the way in which relationships make us feel – particularly if it is someone we know we can trust, who has been there for us and with whom we have a special psychological connection. This is sometimes referred to as a secure attachment relationship. Secure attachment relationships provide a strong foundation, giving you the confidence to work towards personally important goals, safe and secure in the knowledge that there is support available from an established relationship when needed, particularly in times of stress.

People we are strongly attached to are people we want to be close to (physically as well as emotionally). We don't want to be separated from them, and we will often turn to them at times of distress and turmoil. We get support and encouragement from them to tackle new challenges, and the confidence to try out new activities in life. If such a person dies or is lost, say through a break-up, this loss of connection and support is hugely significant and causes major challenges with coping, particularly since it is usually precisely the person who is no longer there who would have been the source of strength and support in this sort of circumstance.

Responses to grief can sometimes be understood by thinking about a psychological theory called attachment theory. Your reactions to a loss now might be influenced by your significant attachment relationships from the past. It is important to understand this aspect of your adjustment and relationships as significant attachment figures are often sought out at times of stress and distress. Complicated grief symptoms are very much focused on the distress associated with separation from the person who has died and also the psychological trauma that has been triggered by the personal impact of bereavement. The links between bereavement and how this triggers efforts to be closer to attachment figures, together with the fact that this is not possible owing to the mismatch with 'the working model' of that person being available and the need to inhibit behaviours fixed on finding the person who has died, are outlined in Figure 2.1. This also shows that in order to adjust to a death there is a need to work towards integrated grief: that is, a point where it is recognized that the attachment figure is no longer available.

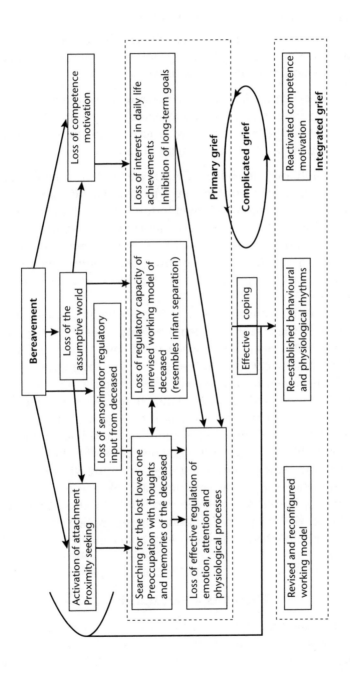

Figure 2.1 Complicated grief pathway based on attachment model

(*Developmental Psychobiology* 47(3): 253–67. Copyright © John Wiley & Sons 2005. This material is reproduced with permission of John Wiley & Sons, Inc.)

Understanding your significant attachments

Think about who the significant attachment figures have been in your life. In your notebook, list the people to whom you have had significant emotional attachments, as below:

- Who have been the key attachment figures in your life?
- How have they helped you in prior times of stress and distress?
- What did you learn about them, yourself and the world as a result of their previous involvement in your life?

During childhood, attachment figures are usually parents, siblings and others who provide care and love. Friends, peers and romantic partners tend to be added to this list during adolescence and into adulthood. Part of understanding your life experience of attachments and separation, as well as identifying how separation through death can be managed, involves taking some time to see whether you can identify any patterns for change or areas you can use to cope.

Changes in attachments result in psychological reactions and also influence the extent to which future attachment changes are significant. Think about times when there have been changes in significant attachment relationships in your life and transitions in attachments more generally, and add these to your notebook.

One of the models of grief is in relation to the revisions of mental models of attachment that take place. If there is some level of stress or threat to the information about an active relationship or attachment, this can trigger a strong desire to be with the person – think about the sort of desires and urges regarding who you want to be with when something upsetting happens. A strong sense of insecurity can result, and behaviour becomes fixed on trying to get in touch with the person. Consider the sort of behaviours that people engage in when there has been a public incident involving loss of life.

Thoughts about suicide

Thoughts of wanting to die can occur in as many as 65 per cent of people after a bereavement, and as many of two-thirds of the people who get these thoughts may have self-destructive behaviour. People with complicated grief symptoms are five times more likely to have thoughts of suicide, a feature that has been reported in adults of all ages but also in young people. Some studies suggest that as many as one in ten people with complicated grief symptoms have made a suicide attempt. This is an example of accommodating the death – seeing suicide as a way of gaining control over the uncontrollable pain and set of reactions. Some people put themselves at risk as a result of neglectful behaviour, or with less regard for risk-taking in general. It is thought that this too might be an example of beliefs that have developed based on helplessness and pointlessness.

You may have noticed that, even if you do not have specific thoughts of ending your life, your behaviour is less concerned with taking care of yourself or you may be acting in a way that could increase the likelihood of accident or death. Does this apply to you? If you have not had such extreme thoughts, the general principle of reducing your self-care may be relevant to your situation.

If you have had any previous experiences in your life of self-harm or suicide attempts and this book has confirmed that you have symptoms of complicated grief then you should speak with a healthcare professional as soon as you can about risk to yourself.

3

How has your grief reaction become complicated?

The first two chapters have outlined the characteristics of grief, acute grief and the way in which complicated grief happens. If you have identified that you have features of complicated grief, then this chapter is where you will start to work on the process of dealing with your distress and confronting thoughts and feelings that you may have been avoiding or pushing away up until now.

This chapter will help you start to learn that it is possible to focus on distressing and painful feelings and that starting to build this into your recovery programme will free your mind, allowing it to zone in on some of the other memories and pieces of information that you have not been able to think about because of the dominance of your loss in your mind.

As I mentioned in the prior chapters, acceptance, adjustment and recovery after a loss do not happen in a single 'proper' way – the path to these outcomes is varied and very individual. Sometimes acceptance, adjustment and recovery require a change in thoughts and beliefs about what has happened; they may require changes in coping strategies, behaviours, relationships or other elements of your life situation.

All the changes that happen relate to someone's overall perspective, the 'story' of the death that has been laid down in mind and memory. Some people who have written about this element of therapeutic work refer to it as working on 'the story of the death'. While many people find this kind of narrative therapy helpful, at a certain stage of grief it can seem inappropriate, even glib. That I should suggest this probably says more about me that it does about the concept itself – it is of course a story – but personally I think that if someone said to me, 'Tell me about the story of the death,' I would think this was minimizing the significance of what had happened. This is an interesting illustration of the importance of the way thoughts influence reactions, and I include it here both by way of explanation and as an illustration of the point that thinking is vital to understanding and promoting recovery.

Writing about the death

Despite what I have just said about 'the story of the death', writing does play a key role in recovery from complicated grief. But it's writing that explores and challenges your established perceptions of what happened rather than the kind that wraps it up in a 'story' to be unchanged for evermore. We all know how such stories can become part of family myth, and how difficult it can be to access the reality of what happened.

Coping more effectively with complicated grief begins when you start to confront and understand all the ways in which focusing on the loss is painful and distressing. This can be done through an exercise that encourages you to write your recollections of the events just before, during and after the death – capturing your thoughts, feelings and memories in as much detail as possible and becoming aware of how your distress is triggered by bringing this into your mind.

To do this exercise, imagine you are back at the time when your loved one died, beginning at the moment that you realized he or she was dead. Write this in the present tense: that is, as if you are writing it at the time you are experiencing, thinking, feeling and reacting to events. Don't be too concerned that you are capturing all the information initially, as there will be other chances to add to this. Indeed, you will need time in which to revise and expand on this first account – it is unlikely to be full and complete in the first draft.

The aim of this work is to capture the perspective you currently have about the death and then, repeating the exercise, to add in more and more details. Remember the importance of memories and how you have linked connections in your mind about the person who has died. These recent loss-related memories are the ones we will be starting with.

Although the first time of writing about the death is likely to be linked with intense distress and grief, the intensity of your emotions will start to diminish when you repeat this exercise and you start to include a wider range of information. You will also be able to use this to support the overall aim of removing the complications to your grieving process. When you feel you have finished reviewing, revising and rewriting, I recommend that you record your account on a digital recorder or smartphone so that you can listen to the description a few times.

This technique was first used in work to help people overcome post-traumatic stress symptoms. It helps to identify the way in which someone's mind has captured the stressful event and, in addition to increasing confidence about being able to confront this, it can be very helpful in highlighting areas where there are gaps in perspective or where specific 'stuck points' might be making it difficult to overcome the personal trauma or to make sense of the way in which part of the event happened.

As I outlined in Chapter 2, many of the complications of adjustment to grief can be understood in terms of the way in which your mind has 'made sense' of what has happened. It is also known that writing about distressing experiences can assist with coping. Sometimes the very act of writing helps get things clearer in our minds. It also may mean spending time thinking about or feeling emotions in relation to an event that we would otherwise not consider for any length of time, or that would quickly be dismissed or avoided completely if it did come into our minds.

Writing down a sequence of events – before, during and after death

The main things to remember are:

- Write this in the present tense (e.g. 'It is 4.30 p.m. and I am entering the room. It smells of lavender and I can see John sitting beside Mum. She is looking so grey and pale. I think, "I can't face this, we are really losing her"').
- You will feel distressed in working through this exercise. If you need to stop and have a break, draw a line across the page and come back to it later.

Adding more details

The next section consists of questions to help you consider whether there might be additional elements of your recollections and perspective on the death that need to be added in your next draft.

- Have you included details of all the emotional reactions that you were having at the time?
- Have you slipped into the past tense at any point in your writing?
- Do you explain what you are thinking when events are happening?
- Have you included details on the physical sensations that you felt at the time?
- Are there any sights, smells or sounds that you can add into the description?

It is likely that the initial summary of your experience of the death and all the subsequent reactions that have complicated your grief will contain many features that you will want to change or approach differently over time. It is common, for instance, for the first written account to be very much about all the painful aspects of the loss, the intensity of the emotional pain and the way in which this has dominated your life.

Don't rest content with your first draft – though it is a valuable beginning. It takes courage to break through your natural defences and into the pain you felt at the time. I cannot stress enough how much you might feel an urge to skim over this task, to rush it or to include only sketchy details. The description needs to capture intensely distressing content to fully reflect the heartache, tragedy and intense vulnerability that might have been a part of your experience.

When people first attempt this exercise they usually begin with a shorter summary that has nowhere near enough detail for it to be useful material to support their recovery. This is fine – as a beginning. The details of the death and all the linked events will always be upsetting and there will a degree of wanting to avoid this – none of us like to dwell on distressing memories, though that is why it is important to remind yourself of the reason for this. Some of the coping statements below might be helpful if you find your attention wandering and/or you are having thoughts that undermine your commitment or confidence in completing this task.

- I feel like this because avoidance is a part of the complications I have had in my grief reaction.
- The distress is a sign to me that I am not getting over this. I need to stop and come back to this later – it is all right to take this in small steps.

If you find that you are overwhelmed by distress, draw a line under the last section you have written and put your notebook away in a drawer to come back to later. The surge in distress will usually be something that will prove significant. There may be more information for you to expand upon in your description, or it might possibly be a sign that what you were writing about represents a particular emotional 'hot spot' or a 'stuck point' in your thinking about the death, your grief and reactions to this. There is more about stuck points later in this chapter.

Grief and its related feelings will always be a part of your life. The aim of this work is not to remove or get rid of these feelings, but to make it possible for you, in time, to recall the circumstances of the death and to experience the grief and distress without the painful longing and yearning and the obsessive rumination over details. And eventually it aims to guide you into thinking about how your connection with the person might be channelled into your future plans for a life without him or her.

Try writing your account over again, building in any more details that may have come to mind after considering some of the issues above.

Although it may seem initially that all your emotions are negative, there may be times when you have some positive feelings related to your experience – such as thinking that the pain and suffering of the deceased is no longer an issue. If there is anything like this that comes to mind, write it down so you can refer to it later as part of your plan to restore some balance and quality of life. If this seems like an alien concept as your grief has been so negative and all-consuming, then come back to it at another time.

When your summary is complete

Once you have completed your summary, read over it again and note down any new points or content that come to mind. Now, if you can, read it aloud. This will help you to focus on the content of what you have written, particularly if you can also visualize this as you read. In your notebook, try to keep a record of the distress levels that you experience as you read this out. Use a 0–100 scale where 0 stands for no distress and 100 for the utmost distress.

You should now have a written account of the details of what happened before the death, around the time of it and afterwards. It will be written in the present tense and in as much detail as you can recall, taking account of the thoughts, feelings, senses and behaviours as they happened. You will now also have some distress ratings that have been added to this to give a sense of the parts of your memories of the death and grieving experiences that are most closely linked with continuing distress.

It is important that you now do something that will promote a sense of reward for yourself, in acknowledgement of how difficult this just-completed task has been. Take time off and distract yourself with another activity that will occupy your mind and give you some relief and respite from the detailed examination of distressing memories. Don't be too concerned if you feel very tired after this exercise; it can be tiring to focus on things that you would usually avoid.

Facing up to avoidance

Although often your urge will be to avoid thinking of what happened, the following are a well-known series of exercises that will help you face this and develop ways of dealing with the range of negative emotions that you will experience.

Now that you have a description of events that are written down, this can be used to help you with urges to avoid painful feelings. Make a commitment to read over (or, if you can, record on a digital recorder or smartphone and listen to) the account of what has happened. Do this every day and really try to focus on the memories, without pushing them from your mind. As well as helping you confront your emotional reactions, this can help with acceptance and is a further way of acknowledging the importance of the person who has died.

Every time you think about the sequence of events, the chances are that you will learn something new, or discover an aspect of your reactions to the death that you had not noticed or acknowledged before. Make sure there is space at the end of each writing session for you to notice and note down any new elements that have emerged as you revise and add to the description.

Exercise 3.1

Keep a record of the dates and times that you add to your draft, and your notes of what happens in terms of your urge to avoid this. Here's a suggested format to copy into your notebook:

Date	Time	Notes (including distress and urge to avoid)

You will now have a written summary of everything that has happened since the death, up to the present. This includes details of your thoughts, feelings, sensations, reactions and responses to events. You will have an idea of the elements that are most distressing for you, and the areas where it has been most difficult to get your head round what happened. You should have a clearer idea of how you reacted, and you have also perhaps identified elements of recent experiences that were not uppermost in your mind – probably because your mental intent was geared to pushing this from your mind, trying not to experience the full amount of distress or emotional pain involved.

It is thought that the more time you spend thinking about, refining and reading the details of the sequence of events, the closer you will start to feel to the person who has died. This idea can seem difficult to accept when you first think about it – you might wonder how writing something down can lead to this important type of change. Simple as it sounds, however – almost too simple – it does involve facing and managing a very painful, important and complex aspect of your life.

If you have been spending some time on this work, it is important at the end to balance yourself by regulating your breathing, and taking a few minutes to close off the work, perhaps by planning something completely different to occupy your mind.

There have been two important elements to revisiting your recollections of the death. The first involves getting you to add more information to your draft as it came to mind, according to the guidelines and questions at the start of this chapter. The other is in relation to the benefits that have been shown to result from this repeated revisiting of your perspective. Repeatedly bringing it to mind helps reduce the avoidance, and boosts your confidence that you can approach the distressing memories without the need to avoid them. It also means that you are starting to have connections to all the elements of your recent experiences, even the very upsetting aspects. Remember that much of what is involved with overcoming complicated grief is related to restoring the natural psychological recovery and healing mechanisms that have become blocked or stuck in your case.

As you read and/or listen to this account of events, it can also start to help you identify thoughts and beliefs that are a part of your overall reaction to your loss and grief.

- Notice the emotions linked with the most distressing recollections.
- Notice the other thoughts you have when you read over what has happened. What comes to mind? What is most distressing about this and what has this meant to you about the person, his or her death and the way your life has been changed?
- Did any new information come to mind that you might want to build into this work, to better understand what has happened?

Notice any differences between how you felt at the time and how you feel now as you are reading this out loud. Is there any difference in the intensity of the emotions that you feel as you read this for the second and third time? If so, what do you make of it? What could the implications be for the process of you coping and recovering?

Don't expect that there will be dramatic changes: the idea is that reversing some of the avoidance promotes a sense of you initially being a little less uncomfortable in thinking and speaking about the death. This is then built on as you feel able to repeat the process, perhaps focusing a little more on the memory.

Now look over your reactions. The most important part is to start looking at some of the thoughts that might be getting in the way of the natural healing and mourning process. Here are some observations that people have made when they have reviewed their detailed written description:

- 'I did not do enough for her.'
- 'He died without knowing how much I love him.'
- 'I can't tolerate not knowing how much or if she suffered.'
- 'It was unfair how he died.'
- 'I don't know if she is at peace.'
- 'Is it right for me to enjoy life without him?'

Now that you have a good understanding of everything that is in your memory in relation to the grief, you can begin to use this as part of helping yourself respond differently to grief. Although you have identified all the elements of the death experience that are in your memory, chances are that these are jumbled in your mind and may not fully explain all the ways in which these memories have had an impact on your feelings and thoughts about life.

Reviewing what you have written for stuck points

The written content that arouses the highest level of distress is often linked to 'stuck points' – aspects of what you have experienced that are difficult to make sense of or 'get your head round'.

These stuck points are areas where there is a conflict between old ways of thinking and the painful reality of what you have had to face as a result of the death and your reactions to it. For example, if you believed that the lost person would be around all your life, or that the person's 'healthy approach' to life meant that he or she would outlive you, then these beliefs are clearly at odds with the death. When you are reviewing what you have written about grief and your experiences after the death, try to notice when you are using words like 'blame', 'fault', 'never', 'always'. These can also be clues to the stuck points in your experience. However, it would not be possible to list all the ways in which there can be these sticking points between old belief systems and the beliefs or thoughts that have become the focus of your daily life since the death.

Look at the latest version of what you have written and circle the sections where you feel you are still struggling to make sense of what happened, or that you cannot get your head around. For each circled section, use some of the questions below to help you identify what the stuck point might be. This can often help clarify ways in which your perspective on the death or your reactions to it are complicating the natural mourning process.

- What is the most difficult aspect of this part of your experience for you to get your head round?
- When you focus on this, what does it mean to you about the world you are now living in?
- When you think about living the rest of your life with this way of viewing events, what practical problems and challenges does this confront you with?
- Since this happened, what theories have you tended to have about why things have turned out like this?

Now review the final written summary of the events and then use your notebook to record areas where you think there are stuck points.

One step at a time

In this chapter, you were encouraged to spend time thinking about and writing an account of the death, first by writing as much as you could, describing this as it actually happened and then, through revising and expanding, adding in more information as it came to mind. Rating the distress helped you to see that it is possible to focus on upsetting aspects of your grief reaction. This also helped you get used to the idea of thinking more about the person who has died, and perhaps slightly more dispassionately, thus making it easier to start building up a wider range of thoughts, memories and feelings about this person. Conversely, if you were not able to start facing the distressing memories of the death, it's likely that this would overwhelm later attempts to cope with your grief and to start rebuilding your life once more. Bear in mind, then, that confronting the actual death is very much a first step and no one is asking you to do more at this stage. Psychologically, however, it is an enormously important step and cannot be skipped. If you do not spend time listening to, reading and re-reading your account of the death, future attempts to cope with your grief are likely to be undermined by preoccupation, fear and the generally distracting effect of your mind bringing you back to your original 'default' position of the distress related to the death. Remember, the aim is to change this initial perspective.

When people are receiving treatment based on techniques similar to the ones in this book, this often involves repeatedly focusing on the distressing aspect of memories in the safe environment of a therapist's office – which can help with the fear subsiding and changes happening in the way that the memories are linked with feelings and prior memories in the person's mind. Approaching this work on your own can be more challenging, though remember that you need to take this gradually and that small steps towards recovery are all that are required each time you face the challenges of the grief. Although it may be difficult for you to acknowledge or believe at the moment, the feelings that you have been experiencing will become less intense with time.

4

Monitoring the impact of grief

So far, I have outlined the way in which reactions to grief can become complicated, and stressed the importance of providing a framework for you to unpack all the details from your mind and memory about the circumstances of the death, expanding on what you were thinking and feeling at that time.

The next crucial element of supporting your recovery is to consider in detail on a day-to-day basis the impact of the grief on your quality of life. This will provide a way of identifying areas where things have become stuck, or where you need to implement new tactics to allow the natural psychological healing processes to resolve your grief.

When you are in the middle of a life experience that triggers strong emotions like grief, anxiety, panic and anger it can be really difficult not to get trapped in a cycle of 'thought paralysis'. This is when the same thought becomes fixed in your mind and influences almost everything that you experience. Your stream of thought does not move but stops, often at the most traumatic point in an experience. This in turn influences your behaviour and coping responses. The previous chapters have looked at your memories of what has happened and stuck points, supporting you in being able to think in ways that will help your recovery. This chapter now examines the wider impact on your life since the point when the death occurred.

This chapter is divided into sections, first considering the overall impact of the grief on your life, and breaking this down into factors such as feelings, thoughts and behaviours. Looking at the main feelings that you have been experiencing will help with further sections on thinking and links to changes in behaviour, particularly with any avoidance pattern that might have developed as your grief reaction has become complicated.

In the same way that you wrote down a summary of the events relating to the death, this chapter will help you outline and summarize the impact. You can then monitor this over a week or two, using it to identify areas where recovery and psychological restoration is more challenging.

You may well have been feeling that you need to be strong for other people, and that this could mean that you have not been able to face up to the reality and finality of the death that has occurred. Thinking of your lost loved one in the past tense might be provoking extreme negative reactions that can trigger panic or other strong feelings. You may have been trying not to think about the impact on yourself, hoping that you will be able to retain a sense of yourself that is unchanged.

Think about all the ways in which the death has changed your life. This may be something you have not considered before, but now make a conscious effort to take your mind back to elements of your life that were present before but are not a part of it now. Make sure that you include feelings and emotions you have been experiencing. As you may remember from Chapter 2, where I outlined what happens in complicated grief, emotional responses to grief can include yearning, rumination, longing, bitterness, anger and a tendency towards preoccupation.

This will help you to think about which sticking points are complicating your reaction to grief, and to identify problematic thoughts that are blocking adjustment to grief. It can also provide ideas for ways of thinking about the deceased person's life and its link with your life (both in the past and moving into the future) that are focused less exclusively on the death and its lead-up. Ultimately you will be able to revisit the statement you will be writing from this chapter and, I hope, be able to recognize the importance of the impact and incorporate this into a view of the experience that helps you build a future less dominated by grief.

For this task to be effective, you will need to plan a time and place where you can write thoughtfully, without being interrupted or distracted. This might not be easy if you have caring or other demands, or are scared that if you let go of your avoidance the emotion will overwhelm you. So, first think about which factors might get in the way of you spending some time writing about this – this is important as so much of the self-help approach outlined in this book involves taking time to write about painful and distressing aspects of your reactions and response to grief. Your overall adjustment may also make it likely that you will try to avoid this exercise. It might assist with motivation with this to make a start on the planning exercise to begin with, and think of it as a series of small steps.

Planning what to write

The following checklist outlines the sort of areas that you may want to cover in your drafting of the statement of the impact the death has had on your life:

- Feelings
- Thoughts
- Behaviour
- Relationships
- Avoidance coping
- Work
- Family
- Interests
- Health.

In your notebook, make some notes against each of these headings, setting down the biggest differences in your life now compared with before your bereavement or loss.

Now outline all the ways in which your life has been affected by the death and all the loss that this has encompassed. Thinking about the initial questions below will help you to begin to construct your statement about the impact loss and grief have had.

- How has life changed since your loss?
- What never happens now as a result of the change?
- What has been the most noticeable change for you?
- What have others commented on that is different now?
- What do you miss most about your life before the loss?
- What has surprised you most about your thoughts and feelings?
- How has this had an impact on the way that you think about yourself, your relationships, your life, quality of life and the world in general?

The following list of life domains will help you think about the impact of the death on your life, ensuring that when you write, you will be considering the impact in a way that encompasses all the areas of your life. This might be the first time that you have considered the reaction in some of these life domains, meaning that this writing could take longer or that you will need time to think about it – particularly difficult if it is painful – before writing.

- Pain and discomfort
- Energy and fatigue
- Sexual activity
- Sleep and rest
- Thinking, learning, memory and concentration
- Self-esteem
- Bodily image and appearance
- Mobility
- Activities of daily living
- Use of medicines and medical aids
- Use of alcohol, tobacco and other drugs
- Communication with other people
- Capacity for work and hobbies
- Personal relationships
- Practical social support
- Caring for other people
- Freedom, physical safety and security
- Home environment
- Work satisfaction
- Financial resources
- Use of health and social care services
- Opportunities for acquiring new information and skills
- Participation in and opportunities for recreation/leisure activities.

Avoidance

Remember, your mind is pre-programmed to go into avoidance mode when experiencing grief. Unblocking paths to psychological recovery often involves identifying any such avoidance. Avoidance can happen on many levels – for example, behavioural avoidance in terms of avoiding situations, places or other people.

- What situations have you been avoiding?
- Which people have you been avoiding?
- What are the benefits of avoidance for you?
- What helps when you avoid thinking about your grief and feelings about grief?
- What helps when you avoid any reminders that could trigger the grief?

Avoidance often occurs because of predictions that the activity being avoided will result in unbearable increases in sadness and yearning for the person who died. If you recognize this, think about the ways in which the grief has impacted on your life to make you avoid something. Have you noticed anything that you avoid doing now because of the death?

Avoidance behaviours have been shown to be linked with three themes:

- Avoidance of places and things that are reminders of the death;
- Avoidance of activities that are reminders of the loss;
- Avoidance of situations related to illness or death that might evoke sympathy.

This can involve avoidance of places, houses or even rooms that are linked with the person who has died. Which reminders of the death have you been avoiding?

Features of your grief

The following questions will also help you to start thinking about the impact of the grief on you, your life and personal experiences:

- What did you expect would happen when you experienced the death of a loved one?
- Was this something that you had thought about before?
- Was it something you tended to avoid thinking about?
- Is the situation different from what you would have imagined?
- What have other people been saying to you about how you have reacted to the death?
- Have other people given you any advice about coping? What have you thought about this?
- Do you have specific ideas or have you learned something from

your life to date that influences how you think people should be reacting to a death?

- Have you been able to deal with all the practical tasks that you have encountered after this person's death?
- What are the predominant memories and thoughts you have been noticing about the person who died? It may be that because of the pain of your grief you cannot face thinking about memories, though taking it slowly and in a gradual and controlled way might be helpful.

Recognizing such features of your grief will help you to adjust to your life without the person you cared about. Although you may not think so, there are many things that you already know about your grief – when it is most likely to be experienced, the physical signs and sensations that are linked with it, the sights, sounds and smells that are most likely to trigger it. Can you take a few minutes to become more conscious of all this? Can you think about specific times when you have felt grief? Were all these situations associated with the same intensity of grief? If not, what do you think it was that made the grief more intense at some times than at others?

Beliefs

If religious belief and church attendance were an important part of the life you had before the death, this may be providing you with a sense of comfort and helping you to make sense of the death. Beliefs can provide a framework to understand and react to the death, and the belief that this event is all part of a higher purpose and plan may mean you are less likely to have particular stuck points. In some instances, however, people with strong religious beliefs do get stuck and begin to question how their pain and distress can be part of any intentional plan of a loving God.

Exercise 4.1

Spend some time thinking about the emotions you have been feeling. These could be guilt, anger, shame, fear, hopelessness, anxiety or fear.

Now that you have read more about the ways in which grief can impact on life, are there any other effects that you had not considered before? Jot them down in your notebook.

Writing an impact statement

Now that you have spent some time thinking about the impact of the death on your life, pull all this together in what is called an impact statement. The impact statement contains all the detail that you have considered, with an emphasis on the meanings you have attached to all the changes.

Developing this can often involve a few drafts as you pull together all the important strands of what has happened. Remember that this is different from the writing in the last chapter (which was on the sequence of events). The emphasis now is on thinking more generally about what the biggest changes are in the way you see the world, your life and your future – the ways in which you have tried to make sense of what has happened. Look at how this has changed or strengthened your views about yourself, others and the world in general.

Here's an example.

> The overall feeling for me of what it means to have lost Sarah is that I must have done something to deserve such pain and sorrow. I feel that so much is negative that nothing will ever feel good again. The world is too full of sorrow and pain for anything to mean anything ever again – it is just that other people do not see this. I can't seem to put any energy into anything as I think that it will all come to nothing. My views are bringing down everyone else around me and I can't think of anything positive any more. This means that everything that I had and valued is pointless and there is no hope of ever recovering from this pain and constant misery.

Exercise 4.2

Now have a go yourself. Put a heading in your notebook, 'Impact statement number 1' and try to record the impact the death has had on you.

Looking for stuck points in your impact statement

Throughout this book we've been considering how normal grieving processes have become complicated and have not been able to progress as they are naturally programmed to do. Earlier on, in Chapter 3, when you were revisiting your memory of the death, you looked for points where there was intense distress as clues to where there might be stuck points in your grieving. The same can be applied to the impact statement. Focus on issues that you keep coming back to – themes in your thinking, and areas where it is impossible for you to move on. Think about the times when you have actually used the words 'I'm stuck' or 'I'm stumped' or 'I can't try any more' or similar (think of your own word or phrase here – something that indicates you have given up completely on this, that it's not possible for you to change this on your own). What were you experiencing when you said this? What would have needed to happen for you not to feel stuck or stumped? Is the fact that you are stuck having a negative impact, and are you aware of the disadvantages? As mentioned before, it is thought that stuck points might be related to a mismatch between some of the things that you thought before the death and some of the experiences you have had since the death.

Beginning a grief impact diary

Now that you have identified some aspects of your life where your bereavement has had an impact, think about which elements you need to understand better if you are to truly appreciate and make sense of the way in which your quality of life is changed. Perhaps it is a mood, a way of thinking or a tendency to cope with challenges in the same way. Perhaps it could be all three of these. The next exercise suggests that you start to keep a grief impact diary over the course of a minimum of one and a maximum of two weeks. This way you will be able to confirm the impact that you have noted in this chapter, and possibly identify some new effects that grief is having. It's likely that you will also notice some patterns about the impact of grief on your life.

Note down how intensely that you have been feeling emotions. This will help you work out whether there are any patterns in terms of your feelings, but will also help you notice which feelings you are having more often. Note down whether you have noticed the same reactions in yourself to different events. For example, do you have similar reactions to hearing a piece of favourite music, taking a familiar walk, e.g. to the shops or the station, or hearing the post arrive?

Monitoring your thoughts, feelings and behaviour for a couple of weeks can be helpful in identifying more details of the impact of your grief on your life. This can in turn be helpful in developing a revised impact statement that incorporates new information.

Now select the main impact you have identified. Pay attention to the way in which this comes up day to day for you – in your emotions, behaviours and what you spend time thinking about. Do this for at least a week to see if you can identify any other ways in which your way of viewing things has changed – remember to look for what you are having most trouble making sense of. Exercise 4.3 shows how such a diary might look.

Exercise 4.3

The main impact on my life is that . . . *nothing I do will make anything feel positive.*

When this happens, I will note what I am doing, how I feel and anything else going through my mind.

Impact event	Feeling	Behaviour	Other thoughts
Post arrives	Despair	Put it in drawer	More negative news
Mark's birthday	Anger	Make excuse	I can't be more positive

This monitoring shows that . . . *my stuck point is: being able to get through each day without problems and negatives dominating my thoughts. I seem to be stuck on the idea that life will always be full of problems.*

The next chapter begins to expand upon the ways in which stuck points influence recovery and how you can begin to think about other ways of approaching these dilemmas caused by complicated grief.

5

Managing the impact of grief on your life

Now that you have considered in some detail how grief has affected your life, and identified stuck points, you can begin to look at specific tactics that can be used to support changes in your feelings and encourage the natural psychological recovery process.

Having effective support

It is a truism that 'talking to someone' helps to 'get it off your chest', but why exactly is this? What seems to happen is essentially a clarification and sorting process that can be of enormous benefit in ordering the often jumbled, confused and stuck thoughts of the person with complicated grief. And of course there's the simple human factor – the benefits of sharing. It is important to keep in mind that grieving and mourning is a natural process and that most of the time the outcome will be a deepening in humanity and connectedness with emotion as a result of the mourning process.

Different psychological theories have attempted to explain why emotional expression is helpful as part of mourning and adjustment to a death. It is generally accepted that expressing feelings can help with the way in which the information is stored within memory. This helps memory and mental representations of the person who has died to be established in new ways – particularly as the reality of what has happened is acknowledged. Expressing and feeling emotion without avoidance will help with the acceptance of the reality, too.

If emotional expression or openly talking about the death and its impact on you has not yet happened, then it could be that your memories of the events leading up to the death have been stored in a jumbled and fragmented way. This is common when grief reactions have become complicated – there seems to be no order or logic to what has been happening.

When you are able to, expressing emotions and talking about the triggers for emotion can help to get elements of your memory sorted into some form of order. You will have no doubt heard people say things like, 'Let me get my head straight' or 'I need to talk about that more to get my head round what you are saying.' Talking about events is a way of helping your mind process what has happened, helping you 'get your head around it' – understanding all that has happened and the links between this and the way you feel. Talking is also important in that it helps you to realize you can experience grief in a relatively safe way – although it will still be painful and upsetting, it is possible to do this without it becoming overwhelming and out of control.

Has there ever been a time when you have said something back to someone else, just to make sure that you have remembered or understood what he or she was saying? This helps you ensure that all the elements of what has happened are stored in the right sequence and are correct. It is very similar to what I have been saying in relation to the griever's need to try to order and understand what has happened. When an event creates strong emotion, you might not have been able to pay attention to everything that was happening, and it is only when you start to talk about this again that every element of the experience comes to light. The same kind of thing happens at times when you have a positive emotional experience such as that commonly associated with a celebration – it is often in the days and weeks afterwards that you are fully able to appreciate it, when you revisit and talk over what happened, sometimes recalling and reliving certain newly remembered elements of the events.

This was part of Exercise 3.1, where you were revisiting and explaining what happened after the death. It can also be used for other elements of your experience where things feel confused or jumbled, or where you find it difficult to put the event into words in a way that makes sense or outlines why it still has an emotional hold on you.

It can be difficult to accept support from other people if you have been thinking that they cannot possibly understand what you have been experiencing. I suggest now that you consider the ways in which other people have been reacting to your experience of grief. When you have thought about this, write down some of the reactions and think about which aspects of the reactions have been helpful, and which less helpful. If some people have had their own difficulties with grief (some of your support network are likely to have had distress and grief about the same death that you are grappling with), perhaps this may suggest the need for you to increase contact with other people who can be more supportive.

As you work through the exercises, bear in mind that although you are doing this work alone, you will probably still need people. Indeed, you may find that being alone with this work accentuates your feeling of isolation, and in this case do consider asking someone to spend some time with you. A close friend or family member might even be able to help you with some of the questions, or at least with getting started on them – this may be especially helpful if you have always been used to having your lost loved one help you like this. People don't always know how much support to offer after a bereavement, so do explain how much of a challenge it is proving to be on your own. Most people will want to help, being available on the telephone or through a webcam as well as popping in now and again. At this stage it might be helpful to remind your friends that what you actually need is companionship in grief, and maybe help doing these exercises, rather than well-meant distractions such as going out for coffee, which you may not yet be up to. Some people may also be keen to hurry the grieving process along, for instance offering to sort out the deceased's effects, which you may also not be quite ready for yet. As was said before, grief goes at its own pace. Ask such people to revisit this in a month or two.

Common emotional responses linked with grief

Continuing grief can be frightening in its intensity, sometimes generating further so-called 'secondary emotions' such as guilt, anger and regret. Think about the main emotions that you have been experiencing as well as grief.

Exercise 5.1

Use the mood list below to help you think about the emotions that might be linked with your grief.

Anger	Shame	Guilt
Disappointment	Depression	Anxiety
Panic	Irritability	Regret

Are there any others? When you have identified them, write them down and consider how they might be linked.

The emotions that come with grief are often very strong and tend to bring a knee-jerk reaction to avoid and push away. You will probably be quite resistant to any suggestion that you do anything other than avoid them; however, just as you revisited memories of your bereavement in a gradual way, you will find it beneficial to do the same with your emotions. Again, take your time and do this in several shorter sessions, with plenty of time in between to process your emotions, rather than in one long draining session.

Avoidance and the impact of grief

Have you been avoiding people, places or activities? Could this be an obstacle to building resilience and making plans for restoring some sense of balance in your life? Avoidance can get in the way of processing all the feelings linked with your grief, and significantly impairs quality of life. Examples of what you might be avoiding are:

- Spending time in some rooms of your home
- Visiting the cemetery
- Reading cards of sympathy or condolence
- Visiting places you used to visit with your lost loved one
- Listening to favourite music
- Spending time with friends, especially those shared with the person who has died
- Sorting through and disposing of personal belongings and other items.

What are the advantages and disadvantages of avoiding? Avoidance can be a way of keeping your distance from painful and distressing emotions. It works very well in the short term for this purpose.

Researchers who have studied avoidance have defined it as 'the phenomenon that occurs when a person is unwilling to remain in contact with particular private experiences (e.g. bodily sensations, emotions, thoughts, memories, events and the contexts that occasion them' (Hayes and Wilson 2003).

If avoidance is used too much or for too long, however, it can actively interfere with the healing functions of mourning and lead to significant complications. As I mentioned in Chapter 1, this is similar to a physical injury where something interferes with the healing process – for example, where a wound is not kept clean or is not cared for, leaving the wound vulnerable to more trauma or subject to complications such as infection.

I cannot stress enough how important it is to begin to think about doing some of the things that you have been very reluctant or frightened to do. However, this doesn't mean gritting your teeth and flinging yourself into the activity. As with other exercises in this book, it can be tackled in small stages. For example, you might think about visiting the cemetery and take some small steps towards a visit without actually visiting. This might involve driving past a few times and then, if the feelings of distress lessen slightly, stopping at the gate, or driving in for a few minutes without leaving the car.

Exercise 5.2

Thinking about the various discoveries that you have made as you have gone through this book so far, use a page in your notebook to recap on what you have been avoiding and the tactics that you have been using to do this.

Now think about your experiences in terms of bodily sensations, emotions, thoughts, memories and life events. Ask yourself if there are ways in which you might have been avoiding these.

- Bodily sensations I have experienced
- Ways in which I have avoided having these bodily sensations

- Emotions that I have experienced
- Ways in which I have avoided having these emotions

- Thoughts that I experience commonly

- Ways in which I have avoided having or paying attention to these thoughts
- Memories that I have experienced repeatedly
- Ways in which I have avoided confronting these memories

- Events that I would usually have attended or been involved with
- Ways in which I have avoided these events.

Helpful and unhelpful avoidance

As we've seen, modern models of grief allow space for avoidance and say it can be beneficial in terms of providing a respite from grief, to allow you to build up your strength. So how can you tell whether avoidance is helpful or unhelpful?

Helpful avoidance occurs in response to changing circumstances and can be thought of as providing respite as part of a wider picture of grief that is moving towards resolution, reclaiming life without the person. Unhelpful avoidance is more of a stable characteristic and is less sensitive to other reactions and responses. In many respects, adjustment to a death is best thought of in terms of a process that works best if it is grappled with, set aside and later revisited. Seeing adjustment in this way can help you start to appreciate that you may have more control over your grief than you have realized, and that controlling how, where and when you focus on grief can be an important step in restoring balance in your mourning.

Avoidance used to distance us from distress tends to result in ineffective processing of the death and significantly diminishes the capacity to restore a sense of joy and life satisfaction. As listed above, this might be avoidance of visits to the final place of death, reading cards or letters, dealing with personal belongings, talking and thinking about the person, visiting favourite places or engaging in a previously enjoyed shared activity. Indeed, research has shown that avoidance is associated with more severe symptoms of complicated grief. You may not have been seeing it as avoidance and it will be difficult for you to identify it as such.

Your exploration system

Researchers who have examined attachment have noted the importance of the 'exploration system', a system that motivates people towards learning, mastery and performance. This system is involved with learning and recovering from a death. However, it can 'switch off' when there is intense stress or when a separation occurs – and it is often shut down or switched off following a bereavement. The following questions can help you think about whether your exploration system may have been shut down or put on standby.

- Are you able to visit the final resting place of the deceased?
- Have you been able to engage in thinking about or doing the things that you used to do with the person?
- Have you been able to visit the places that you used to visit together?
- What are the common day-to-day reminders that intensify your feelings of loss?
- How do you react when this happens?

Having considered this, do you think that avoidance might be an issue for you? Could this be something that is underlying your complicated grief – something that is ultimately holding you back from the process of recovery?

Ranking distress

The next exercise is ranking the amount of distress associated with life activities, using a rating scale for distress and discomfort. A score of 100 is intense discomfort of the sort experienced when intensely anxious or sad, and 0 is the complete opposite, with no distress at all. 'Distress' is being used here as shorthand for a range of negative emotions that are often associated with grief.

Start by writing down scores of 100, 75, 50 and 0 in your notebook. Against each one, provide an example of events recently where you were aware of being emotionally distressed, like this:

100   When the police officer came to the door to tell me Jim was dead

75   Wandering around the house with nothing to do

50   Going back to work and ploughing through the familiar routine, being aware all day that he was gone – no phone calls, no emails – and that he wouldn't be there when I went back home in the evening

0   Soaking in the bath that time when I forgot for a moment that he was gone.

Exercise 5.3

Now that you have an idea of how the scoring system works, use your notebook to write out all the situations, people and places that you are tending to avoid because of the distress that this would cause you.

1 List all these people, places and situations that you have been avoiding (or enduring with very high levels of distress).
2 Give each one of them a score on the 0–100 scale that you used earlier.
3 Now take them and put them in order from the least distressing to the most distressing.

Think about telling someone close to you that you are planning to work through the exercises in this book, so that you can speak with him or her when you need to get an alternative perspective. You could ask if he or she thinks you may have missed other activities that you have been avoiding.

If your life has been characterized by avoidance of emotional expression, then you will tend to cope with grief in this way as well. Think about previous life events and how you reacted emotionally. Did you tend to express your feelings or were you more inclined to suppress them and try to get on with things, not taking the time to understand the impact of the event on you?

Moving your loved one from your mind to your heart

Remember that the way of overcoming the complications with your grief is to work on loss-focused strategies, and restoration-focused strategies (see page 7). Tackling thoughts, emotions and behaviours with this in mind will help you reach a point where you are in control of the impact of your loss and can work to restore dimensions of your life.

Loss-focused strategies (such as avoiding the pain and distress for less of the time) will help with moving your loved one from your mind to your heart. This can be achieved through the revisiting outlined in Exercise 3.1. Imagining conversations and bringing memories of your loved one to mind through conversation and exposure to pictures can also achieve this, and exercises on exposure to triggers that remind you of the person can be part of this work to experience the full pain of the loss.

The goal is to restore satisfying relationships and activities by identifying plans and goals in relation to self-care and other personally important life goals. This might also include problem-solving and dealing with specific life issues that need to be addressed in order to deal with the impact of grief on your life.

What do you consider your personal strengths to be? Could these be used in the plans and actions that you would like to build into your recovery?

Understanding and coping with psychological reactions to grief can make more sense if you think in terms of regaining a sense of control – sometimes called mastery – with the loss and its impact. Your responses to grief so far (particularly in complicated grief) are your mind's reaction as it strives to gain control over what happened. However, sometimes this reaction is counterproductive and might not support the grieving process in the way it is designed to. So let's look at how certain tactics could be blocking you from restoring this sense of mastery, and why loss-related thoughts and experiences may dominate.

Understanding memory networks

As mentioned in Chapter 1, traumatic experiences are thought to lead to the development of a fear network that can in turn lead to escape mechanisms and avoidance. Following a bereavement, this fear network can be thought of as being made up of all the various stimuli and responses that are linked with the grief. Anything that is linked with the event can then trigger the fear memory, meaning that information from the network can come into consciousness; it is this that may be responsible if you are getting regular unwanted and intrusive thoughts about the death and the grief.

So, as well as dwelling specifically on your memory of the death, it is important to think about your life in general. We all have a strong need to determine what happens to us in life, to feel competent and to have a sense of connection and relationship with other people, in order to enjoy a good level of mental health and wellbeing.

It may take time, and more than one session, before you can come up with any answers, but try to consider these questions:

- What provides you with a sense of connection to other people?
- What gives you the feeling of being good at something?
- What were your long-term life goals and dreams?
- What sort of activities tended to bring you a sense of satisfaction before?
- What is the sort of goal or plan that would be satisfying to you – something that had deep meaning for you or was dear to you?
- Is there something that would give you a sense of excitement or anticipation?

Thinking in these terms may seem strange, and a betrayal of the person who has died. They are, after all, an admission that life goes on without that person. But try not to give in to apathy and hopelessness. Try and sit with the questions for ten minutes, thinking about them. Note any reactions – you may experience undefined feelings at first, rather than thoughts. Stay with these until something more definite emerges.

When you are ready, take the answers to these questions and write them down in as much detail as possible. They can be used to start creating your personal commitment to restoring some balance in your life. They are informed by the sense of connection that you have built with the person who has died but, importantly, they are also informed by the connections you will need to build in the future in order to fulfil your potential and improve your quality of life.

It is important to include this as part of an overall approach to dealing with grief, as it will help generate hope and enthusiasm for the future. If you can begin to experience some more positive emotions, this will help your recovery from the complications of grief, as well as providing you with a strong base to keep going with other challenging and difficult work that relates to the grief therapy (and any other life difficulties or challenges that might occur along the way).

Setting goals for the future

- If you could wave a magic wand and make the grief more manageable in your life, what sort of things would you want for yourself?
- What are the things that you valued in life before? When did you have a sense that you were involved in an activity that was an important part of your values?
- When you have identified something that you think you can work towards, it will be important to plan for this, thinking about what would be signs of progress, identifying ways of keeping motivated and committed to this and thinking in advance of some of the things that might get in the way of the goal.
- Are there people that you would want to tell about this plan or goal that you have set yourself?

The answers to these questions should give you some idea of activities you will find it helpful to incorporate into your way of thinking, behaving and living generally, providing a more balanced set of experiences to counteract the dominance of fear and distress that is constantly activated by fear and by memories of the death.

Understanding your range of feelings

You are likely to have a wide range of emotions in response to your bereavement. Do you fully understand and appreciate the range of feelings? What would happen if you paid attention to these for a few days? Have you been experiencing any anguish? Dread? Regret? Anger? Shame? Relief?

For each of the emotions, start to think about:

- Which past events are upmost in your mind when you are experiencing this feeling?
- Are there stuck points that you could spend some time thinking about (instead of avoiding), identifying what you could change in order to restore previous elements of your life?

Guilt

All emotions are generated by some level of interpretation or judgement. When people feel guilt this is usually because they think there is something they have done that they 'should' not have, or something they 'should' have done that they have omitted to do. You may be in two minds about whether your actions have actually had a bearing on what is making you feel guilty. It can be a good idea to talk to someone who was not closely involved. This can help you decide whether you have acted in a way that is in fact 'blameworthy' and whether it was your intention for events to turn out in the way that they did.

Guilty feelings are often associated with judgements that are being applied to your role in a sequence of events – usually that you have broken an important rule or acted in a manner that has violated personally important rules or values for you or other people.

- What is it that you think you did wrong?
- What important belief or personal value do you think you did not live up to?
- Are you focusing on something that has happened to you unfairly or unjustly, or that you did not deserve?

Consider carefully whether you have actually acted in a way that is 'wrong' or intentionally set out to violate values that are important to you or other people. Maybe you did not intend the outcome to turn out as it did, and your review of events leads you to conclude that your actions were in fact well intentioned. Could you be over-estimating the amount of control that you had in the situation? Also think about all the other factors that may have influenced the situation. Was everything completely within your control? Was it really something you were able to influence at the time? Were any other factors involved? Did others make decisions or have an influence on what was happening at the time?

While it is important to spend time focusing on grief-related emotions, identifying and changing thoughts that could be fuelling these, it is also important to use the insights and learning from this time to make a plan. What does your plan need to be for coping and responding to the guilt that you have identified?

Exercise 5.4

Now think about planning in positive actions and plans, using the word 'if'. *If* your grief were at a more manageable level that it is at the moment,

- what would you be wanting to happen in your life?
- what would be happening day to day?
- which activities would you be doing that, at present, you are not doing because they would remind you that your loved one has gone?

For each of these, how desirable would it be to reintroduce this activity into your life?

This exercise helps you examine how far you may have been putting restrictions on your quality of life – for example, not swimming or going for country walks because this is something you used to do together. Working through these questions can help restore missing elements of your life, or at least enable you to become more aware of them; it also helps with the continuing processing of emotions and information about the final nature of the death.

It is all right to feel relieved after someone has died. This can lead to guilt, even if with one part of your mind you know that death was a release, and that it was 'time' for the person to go, for example in the case of prolonged illness. Guilt may be just one of a complex range of emotions, and it can be confusing to experience positive and negative emotions at one and the same time. But it is also all right – even expected – to feel confused. Allow yourself to feel a range of emotions; try not to cause more challenges by being self-critical or analysing the reasons for them.

Think of the emotions being triggered not so much by the death itself but more by your emotional response to the experiences that followed. You may feel sad and anguished that you will never have the chance to speak to the person, or feel him or her next to you again. At the same time, you may also feel relief that you no longer have to worry about what is going to happen next, or that the telephone is going to ring with more bad news, about the progression of his or her illness, for example. Your recovery will start when you accept it is all right (and expected) for you to have a range of positive and negative emotions within a short space of time. Experiencing these feelings is the first step towards restoration of your life, though it is also acceptable and expected that this will not make sense to you.

It is important to identify activities that provide some positive experiences and to invest time in relationships (either ones that you have been avoiding or new ones).

Anger

If you have been feeling angry, do now think about where the anger is directed. Who are you feeling angry with? Anger is often directed at people who are perceived to have removed control, or to have created a sense of helplessness. You might be angry at medical staff involved with the care and treatment of the person who has died, or the emergency services who were in attendance at the time of the death. You might be angry at the reactions of other family members. Sometimes the anger that you are experiencing is directed towards these people, though when you allow yourself time to identify its source you will notice that the anger is more complex that it appeared at first.

It could be that your anger is directed at society or government or a higher force, such as God. Anger to do with the actions of other people or at 'the world' in general is common. If you have been feeling angry, try to work out who and what this has been directed towards.

Control in daily life

No-one has complete control over the events that happen to them in life. Some of us might have beliefs that emphasize the importance of control, or we may fool ourselves into thinking that we have more control over events than we actually do. Although you may not believe or experience it, it is important that you remind yourself that you are not completely helpless and that you are able to influence both the way in which things happen and your reactions to events. It might not feel like this, but remember that feeling something is not the case is not the same as it being true. If you have difficulty thinking about this in a way that helps you to accept that you have some control or influence, consider the following exercise.

Exercise 5.5

Select a day and during the course of that day make a note of all the decisions you make. List these in your notebook.

Now answer these questions:

- What have you been feeling helpless about?
- What are your options?

You don't need to have total control in order to have control or influence over outcomes or situations. Sometimes it is tempting to think about control in these all-or-nothing terms. You may have been telling yourself that you should have been able to deal with this yourself, or maybe you have been labelling yourself in unhelpful ways that, in addition to causing you distress, result in you being less able to cope with the demands you have been facing. Would it help you to remind yourself that some events in life are too overwhelming and huge to be handled alone?

You and your future

While you will want to do all you can to retain a deep sense of connection with the deceased person, it is just as important that you really think about your life. If you were not experiencing so much distress and turmoil, what would have been your goals or plans? Perhaps there was something that you and the person who has died were planning to do.

Consider these questions:

- What are three plans or goals that you want to make?
- For each one, how will you know that your plans are developing as you want them to, and that you will meet the goal?
- What are the things that you worry would get in the way of meeting the goal or making the plan a reality?
- Is there someone who can help you with each of the plans to make them a reality?

When you think about all that you have been through, what do you think your main reactions have been in relation to yourself and your future? It may be that you cannot even begin to think about what the future could be like without the person who has died. If this is the case, it might be helpful (in the longer term) to think about the plans that you would have had for your future several months or years before the death happened. Write down what you would have said if someone had asked: 'What are your plans for yourself and your future?'

Maybe the shift in perspective that can happen after a death has completely altered your views on the future. You might feel that the future is completely shattered, and that where there were once ideas and hopes for the future, now nothing could ever seem possible. You might feel that planning for the future is not appropriate or timely for someone who is adjusting to a death. Asking yourself, 'What are my plans?' could be at odds with personal rules and beliefs that, when grieving for someone else, your emphasis should not be on personally motivated goals and a way forward.

Do I need medication?

The intensity of the grief that you are experiencing can be treated using medication, but this is something you should discuss with your GP. Medication can be effective even if several months have passed since the death. Currently, though, there is no medication specifically for complicated grief, and perhaps many people deep in grief would prefer not to have their feelings medicated in this way even if it were available.

Some research has shown that taking antidepressant medication at the same time as working on the issues outlined in this book, as part of a therapy, results in a greater improvement in symptoms. Medication can make it more likely that painful and distressing psychological symptoms can be addressed in therapy, or through exercises such as those outlined in this book. In one study, people taking medication were twice as likely to be able to complete the psychological treatment for the complicated grief symptoms that they experienced. This could be related to the impact of medication on sleep, motivation or mood symptoms in general, making it more likely that greater benefit will be gained from the psychological intervention components. Research trials demonstrate that the symptoms of depression tend to improve more than the grief symptoms, though they do improve in the order of 50 per cent from before the medication was started. The research continues; while medication is probably not for everyone, it may provide some people with just enough of a lift to enable them to work on their other grief-related problems and start to re-engage with life.

6

Identifying and conquering problem thoughts about grief

'I will not be able to manage without him', 'Nothing will ever be the same again', ' I will never experience a positive feeling again' and ' There is no solution' are some examples of problem thoughts that may be linked with your complicated grief.

This chapter will look at specific thoughts that might be serving to maintain your thinking and attention on loss and grief, making it difficult for you to get your life back and plan for your future. People's thinking can change after a death. The grieving process entails a whole process of new and often harrowing thoughts, which can become an ingrained part of your thinking even without you realizing it. To a certain extent, of course, these thoughts are vital in helping you assimilate the reality of what has happened and the finality of the loss. But, in complicated grief, if left to themselves such thoughts can interfere with your progress.

Dealing with such thoughts can really help the adjustment to a death, progressing to the point where you can cope with the pain and distress of loss, and build on your new understanding to restore elements of your life that provide a sense of meaning and personal fulfilment. This will help you to gain acceptance of the death, and to discover ways in which you can integrate the pain into a wider set of memories that are connected to other aspects of your life – and to build new memories and experiences. These do not cancel out the painful and distressing memories, but provide a balance that allows you to cope and manage feelings as part of a more open acknowledgement that, although the pain and distress of loss and grief can be overwhelming, there is a chance of beginning to experience positive emotion once more.

Now that you have a sense of some of the ways in which your thinking has been altered as part of your experience of grieving, it can be easier to set about changing this. This is important as the way that you think determines how you will react to mourning and recovery – which coping mechanisms you use, what you give your attention to, and how you plan your day-to-day activities. One of the most common problems is developing a series of thoughts that are designed to create an emotional distance from your feelings and to maintain avoidance of events, memories and people that remind you of the loss.

If it is not possible to gain this level of acceptance, it is possible for grief-skewed thinking to rewrite the history of the death from a highly negative perspective. That is, you interpret the death to match beliefs about the world that are extremely negative and resistant to change, placing yourself at risk of serious levels of clinical depression and helplessness. You may end up blaming yourself for the trauma – 'If only I had been stronger about telling him to go to the doctor', for instance – causing intense guilt and preoccupation about what should have happened to stop the pain and grief from happening in the first place. This is a form of hindsight, where you look back on events as if you had known the outcome in advance.

Secondary emotions

Identifying problem thought patterns about grief can be easier when you distinguish between emotions that are part of the healing and adjustment process linked with grief, and those that are secondary (sometimes called 'manufactured'). When grief becomes complicated, it is often because of thinking patterns that lead to secondary or manufactured emotions – for example, when guilt is manufactured or secondary in addition to grief and sadness linked with loss.

In some circumstances, there can be an extreme alteration in beliefs to the point that the beliefs generate extreme intense emotions such as panic or hopelessness. Here the grief-related reactions are generalized by thought patterns that then apply to a range of situations not directly related to the bereavement, death or grief reaction. Thoughts and attention start to bring in other unrelated life factors, linking them with the bereavement experience. This then leads to a general sense of being overwhelmed by emotions and the reinforcement of the self as being unable to control or influence this important dimension of health and wellbeing. This is shown through thoughts like, 'I will never feel happiness ever again' or, 'There is no point in ever again connecting with someone in the way that I did with her.' It's a kind of false logic, if you like, in which the bereavement mood is inappropriately extrapolated into areas that are – or should be – beyond its reach.

As I outlined in Chapter 3, sometimes stuck points are the result of being overwhelmed by emotions, while at other times they are the direct result of specific thoughts that are experienced about grief and reactions to it. If you have experienced the death of several people you are close to, you may already have the belief that the world is unfair and unjust; a further death may then lead to a generalized belief that starts to see everything in this way.

Think about a recent example when you have been thinking about grief and the changes in your life. Concentrate on what the feelings are in response to this and then ask yourself: 'What does still feeling this way mean to me? What does this say to me about myself? Grief? My life? My coping?' When you have asked yourself this, write down some of the thoughts that pass through your mind.

As a way of identifying alternative thoughts to those that are being experienced about the grief, ask yourself:

- What is the evidence to support this idea that I have about this area?
- Is there anything that I can think of that is not supportive of this idea?
- Could my thinking about this be being influenced by my overall level of distress?

You might have already had thoughts about the world being unfair or cruel, and all that the death has done is to reinforce these for you. If you have been thinking about the death as evidence that the world is unfair, random and unpredictable then you will probably believe this more strongly. This could result in you having emotional reactions that mean you don't take chances or opportunities in the future. You may be starting to behave as if your thinking is a fact. Could there be ways in which your current behaviour is being triggered by some of your thoughts about grief?

Thinking about some of the questions that still go round and round in your mind can give you clues to some of the themes that might be in your thoughts, the kind of themes that can cause manufactured emotions (secondary feelings) that then become imposed on the grief itself. Examples of such questions might be: 'How can someone look so well and then be dead within two hours?', 'How come other people can recover from the same infection and he didn't?'

Here are more questions to help you tune into the ways your thinking may have changed through initial coping with death and associated grief:

- How has this person's death changed your outlook on your family and your relationship with them?
- What changes have there been in your view of work and how it fits with your life?
- Has your experience or view of relationships changed?
- How has your view of yourself changed as a result of this death?

You may have been wishing it was you who died, or feeling that it should have been you. This is common when a death seems to have violated personal rules and expectations about the order in which events should happen or the circumstances that should make death more likely. Perhaps the person was younger than you or lived life in a way that meant they took more risks.

Changing your beliefs about the world and events within it

You need to change your beliefs about the world and events within it, because your world has changed as a result of the person's death. You might not know yet how your beliefs need to change, though one thing is certain: if your beliefs do not change in some way, it will be more difficult for you to cope and adjust to what has happened.

Do you think that your beliefs about the world and events in your life have changed? If so, have you strengthened what you have always believed, or have you created new ways of thinking based on what has happened? Think about this and ponder whether it might be linked with your emotions and behaviours.

Some of your thinking about your loss could be unbalanced and may be causing the psychological recovery process to get stuck. This is often linked with the issues that keep coming back, when you feel, 'I can't get out of my head' or, 'I can't get my head round that' or 'It doesn't make any sense to me.' You might have altered your ways of thinking to become more extreme – 'There is no point in investing time in relationships' or 'It's too painful' or even 'There is nothing that means anything any more.' You might be thinking of differences that you could have made or different ways of reacting, as you try to make sense of what happened and fit this into your belief system.

Here are some examples of the sort of the stuck points that can happen after a bereavement. Reading them will hopefully help you identify the possible areas where you have had stuck points after the death:

- Survivor guilt can result in thoughts that, for example, you have no right to feel any happiness or positive emotions because of the death and that you will no longer feel any happiness again.
- You may feel that you have more power and control than is the case, thinking that you could have prevented the death if you had acted in a different way.
- Sometimes hindsight can introduce bias in thinking, with your thoughts becoming fixed on the idea that if only you had done something else then the death would not have happened.
- You may have had experiences where you have been unable to accept the reality of the death, thinking that, 'This cannot be happening' or, in extreme forms, 'He or she isn't dead'.
- You may have been focusing on the idea that your relationship or life situation in relation to the person who has died was so different and unique that, while you acknowledge other people might be able to adjust or cope with their grief, this is not something that will be possible for you, given the uniqueness of your situation.
- You may be thinking that you will never again experience anything like the relationship that you had, that nothing similar or better could ever occur.

- You may be thinking that your life is completely over now.
- You may have noticed that your thinking has been very biased towards all the positives relating to the person who is dead, to the point where you could have been idealizing or even idolizing him or her. It is important to make sure that this is not preventing you from adjusting to the loss of the real person, and to remember that, like any of us, our lost loved ones had their strengths, weaknesses and eccentricities that made them who they were.
- It may be that there were significant strains or problems in your relationship with the person who has died and that the tendency to focus on positives (or think that it is not right to openly acknowledge any faults or problems) could be preventing you from putting that person's life and death into the complete picture, when you could understand your reactions to the death on the basis of all the information available.

Look back over your summary of events and your impact statements to see if there are any new stuck points that you recognize now as a result of thinking some more about this.

Avoidant coping

Beliefs about death are not something that you will be able to describe succinctly or easily. Attempts to make sense of what has happened, as you begin to consider the implications of the death across various aspects of your life, will often be hampered by thoughts and beliefs that 'get in the way'. This can be linked with your predictions about what will happen if you dwell on the grief. For example, some people become concerned that if they dwell on their feelings of grief, these will become overwhelming to the point that they will lose control of their emotions completely. This way of thinking about grief has been shown to result in high levels of what is known as avoidant coping.

As we have seen, coping through avoidance is characterized by a tendency to push unwanted memories, thoughts and emotions from consciousness. Although this tends to work in the short term, it usually leads to more frequent, overwhelming and intense grief afterwards. Coping responses for intense emotion tend to become established in late adolescence and early adulthood. People who experience intense grief as a normal consequence of a bereavement are more likely to run into difficulties if they tend to cope by minimizing or dismissing negative emotions. Could this be happening to you? If it is, what sorts of thoughts have you been having about grief that might be making this more likely?

The coping responses of other significant people in your life can also have a bearing on your own coping strategies. Consider, for example, someone who tends to cope by openly expressing his emotions and, as a way of coping with his grief, does so with a partner whose preference is not to discuss or think about such distress. This scenario can lead to further psychological challenges if the reason for not expressing feelings is labelled negatively.

Some common thoughts that are associated with avoidant coping with grief are outlined below:

- This is horrible, I am never going to get over this.
- I shouldn't be feeling like this now.
- If I focus on how bad I'm feeling, I'll go mad.
- People are sick of listening to me talking about how I'm feeling.
- I need to pull myself together.
- I'm making other people upset.
- People can't keep seeing me like this.

Once you have looked over some of these common thoughts about grief and expressing feelings, think about how this might be contributing to your day-to-day reactions. It is sometimes helpful to spend some time on a recent example where your thinking about grief was of the type outlined above.

When you have fixed an example in your mind, write down who was present, what date and time it was, what was happening and where this occurred. Once you have briefly described this, spend some time examining the thoughts that were passing through your mind about the reasons not to express your grief. Now think about what you did to suppress your feelings, hide them from others or stop experiencing them. This might include examples such as avoiding or escaping from situations where other people are present, pushing all thoughts, memories or content completely out of your mind.

Now that you have identified some of the ways in which you are thinking and the behaviours about grief that are influencing your coping, the following sections will help you to think about the advantages and disadvantages of your current style of coping. They will also provide you with a structure of thinking about other times in your life where you have experienced strong and intense emotion and whether your current way of coping is unique to your current grief or part of a long-standing pattern that you have used with other strong emotions. The ways of handling this will differ depending on how you have coped with strong emotions previously.

Although not always consciously, many people have mental models or images that are associated with what it means to experience and express strong emotions. Think about other people you know, or characters in films and movies where the expression of strong emotion has been a feature. This might involve a recent storyline in a soap opera such as *EastEnders* or *Coronation Street*.

While thinking about this, also pay attention to any examples that come to mind of strong emotional reactions you have witnessed in other people following a bereavement. Once you have written them down, consider whether these other people's reactions might have influenced what you think and the judgements you might make about such strong emotions.

Some people report feeling extremely unsettled by the strength of grief and how, prior to this experience, they had tended to label other people as being weak or unstable. This can trigger a need to search for a way of making sense of the experience, and in some cases can lead to the development of clinically significant symptoms of anxiety and panic, usually linked to either lack of beliefs about self- or emotional expression to explain the reaction.

Moyra was a 39-year-old woman who had previously worked as a paramedic in the British army. She had first-hand knowledge and experience of speaking with army staff who were discharged owing to the development of significant psychological and mental health problems. Following the death of her father, she presented with severe symptoms of panic disorder and, during assessment, disclosed that she believed that anyone who expressed strong emotions of sadness or anxiety was 'weak'. She had always believed herself to be completely in control of all elements of her life, and was unable to accept that her experience of intense grief and uncertainty about the future was not an example of weakness and loss of control. She believed that such weakness would ultimately end up in her being detained under the Mental Health Act as a result of a progressive increase in the intensity of her anxiety and panic. The strength of her belief that expressing negative emotion was a sign of weakness was so intense that she began to explore alternative explanations, e.g. the possibility that she was suffering from a rare endocrine (hormonal) disorder. As her psychological therapy progressed, she began to find it amusing that she would rather have accepted she had a serious physical health problem, and expose herself to medical investigations involving a degree of risk, than accept that it is normal for a human being to experience intense and at times overwhelming emotion after the death of a parent.

The Grief Cognitions Questionnaire

In addition to considering what has been passing through your mind in general, or noticing that thinking is encouraging you to avoid your feelings, it is also possible to better understand your thoughts in relation to grief by completing a questionnaire. The Grief Cognitions Questionnaire (see Table 6.1) assesses what you have been thinking about the death of someone closely linked with you.

Table 6.1 Grief Cognitions Questionnaire

Below are listed different negative beliefs. Indicate the degree to which you agree with each belief, on a scale of 0–5 (0 is 'disagree strongly', up to 5 indicating 'agree strongly').

Number	Statement	Disagree strongly – agree strongly (score 0–5)
1	Since Sarah is dead, I think I am worthless.	
2	I am partially responsible for Sarah's death.	
3	Since Sarah died, I realize that the world is a bad place.	
4	The people around me should give me more support.	
5	I don't expect that I will feel better in the future.	

Number	Statement	Disagree strongly – agree strongly (score 0–5)
6	I have to mourn, otherwise I will forget Sarah.	
7	I see myself as a weak person since Sarah passed away.	
8	If I let go of my emotions, I will go crazy.	
9	I am ashamed of myself since Sarah died.	
10	The death of Sarah has made me realize that we live in an awful world.	
11	My grief reactions are abnormal.	
12	Life has nothing to offer me any more.	
13	I don't have confidence in the future.	
14	As long as I mourn I maintain the bond with Sarah.	
15	My life is useless since Sarah died.	
16	I don't mourn the way I should do.	
17	I should have prevented the death of Sarah.	
18	Many people have let me down after Sarah's death.	
19	The death of Sarah has taught me that the world is unjust.	
20	My life is meaningless since Sarah died.	
21	My wishes for the future will never be fulfilled.	
22	Since Sarah is dead, I feel less worthy.	
23	If I fully realized what the death of Sarah means, I would go crazy.	
24	If I had done things differently, Sarah would still be alive.	
25	Ever since Sarah died, I have thought negatively about myself.	
26	I do not react to this loss normally.	
27	In the future I will never again be really happy.	
28	As long as I mourn I do not really have to let Sarah go.	

Number	Statement	Disagree strongly – agree strongly (score 0–5)
29	People around me should show much more interest in me.	
30	I will never be able to forgive myself for the things I did wrong in the relationship with Sarah.	
31	There is something wrong with my feelings.	
32	My life has no meaning any more, since Sarah died.	
33	I blame myself for not having cared better for Sarah.	
34	The death of Sarah has taught me that the world is a worthless place.	
35	Since Sarah is no longer here, I have a negative view on the future.	
36	If I allowed my feelings to come out, I would lose control.	
37	Since Sarah is dead, I am of no importance to anybody any more.	
38	If I once started crying, I would lose control.	

(Reproduced by permission of Paul A. Boelen, Department of Clinical Psychology, Utrecht University, PO Box 814, 358 TC, Utrecht, The Netherlands)

Exercise 6.1

Copy Table 6.1 into your notebook, replacing 'Sarah' with the name of your lost loved one and noting your responses.

Grief Cognitions Questionnaire subscales

The questions in Table 6.1 fall into nine subscales:

1 Self (items 1, 7, 9, 22, 25, 37)
2 World (items 3, 10, 19, 34)
3 Life (items 12, 15, 20, 32)
4 Future (items 5, 13, 21, 27, 35)
5 Self-blame (items 2, 17, 24, 30, 33)
6 Others (items 4, 18, 29)
7 Appropriateness (items 11, 16, 26, 31)

8 Cherishing grief (items 6, 14, 28)
9 Threatening interpretation of grief (items 8, 23, 36, 38).

When you have completed this questionnaire, you can look at your responses on each of the nine subscales. This can further help pinpoint what thoughts might be underlying your distress or difficulty coping with and restoring elements of your life changed by grief. We will look at each section in turn, outlining some of the thoughts characterized by negative grief-related thinking. Some pointers will be provided to help you begin to think about alternative ways of considering your experience of grief, identifying areas you might wish to think about and discuss with those close to you over the coming weeks.

Self

- Since Sarah is dead, I think I am worthless.
- I see myself as a weak person since Sarah passed away.
- I am ashamed of myself since Sarah died.
- Since Sarah is dead, I feel less worthy.
- Ever since Sarah died, I have thought negatively about myself.
- Since Sarah is dead, I am of no importance to anybody any more.

If you agreed with these items, your scores on the items in this scale will show more negative thinking about yourself, how you are as a person or the way you have reacted. This indicates that your feelings of sadness and depression are likely to have increased, in addition to the grief that you are experiencing. The emphasis on thoughts about yourself will also make it more difficult for you to make sense of your personal world and future life without the person who has died. Your thinking has become concentrated inward and, as a result, you will become less able to think about ways of coping or accessing support that will help you to understand and adjust to your loss. This is also likely to enhance the inward direction of your attention. You can begin to address such thoughts by considering the following questions:

- What would the person who has died say to you if he or she knew that you were thinking of yourself of worthless and weak?

- What aspects of your responses are you seeing as evidence of weakness?
- What other explanations are there for this other than weakness? Is there anything in the first few chapters on grief that shows that this is a recognized part of grief?

The most effective way to address this is to identify any specific negative thoughts you are having (as the questionnaire is only an indication of themes). You can do this by concentrating for a few days on the negative thoughts you have about yourself in relation to the death that has occurred. This will usually be easier when you notice that they occur when your emotions dip negatively – when you feel more sad, anxious or angry.

- What went through your mind?
- What aspect of the death were you reminded of and what did it mean to you that this was coming back to your mind?
- What did it say about you, the world and your life now that you are still feeling like this?

Asking yourself some questions can widen your horizons and open your mind so you are able to think about other perspectives. If there have been previous times in your life where you have thought negatively about yourself, it may help to remember what lessened the distress then. Often when I ask people about this in clinical work, their attention immediately moves to the fact that life before was not like life now, and that the person who is dead was there to support and help. This is of course a fact and a painful reality of death. In order to make a start on coping mechanisms, it can be helpful to think back to the kind of things that were happening and/or what the person who has died would have done to provide respite for distress.

The all-encompassing sense that 'life cannot ever be the same' can become mentally translated into meaning that there will never again be anything positive to experience. Think about this for a moment. If it is true, then what are the implications? Is this what you are saying? Could it be that this thought is acknowledging the painful and permanent nature of the change in your life, but also stopping you from exploring ways in which life might be different both positively and negatively?

Do you know of anyone who has experienced the death of someone? Most of us know of people who have survived such an experience and recovered to the point where they do have positive experiences again. Could you contact such a person in order to talk to him or her about how this happened? Perhaps he or she thought and felt as you do and could share some ideas about how things changed. What have you noticed in people who seem to have survived the loss of someone close?

You might be thinking, 'Yes, but that's different.' Now while that is true in respect of everyone having individual differences in the nature and pathway of their recovery processes, there are some universals in relation to coping and adjustment. It would be very unusual if there were no similarities between you and the thousands of other people who have recovered some of the prior positives within their lives after a bereavement. What might some of the similarities be? How would you find this out?

If you do not know someone personally or do not have enough information about this, could you think about a public event and/or someone who has written about his or her personal adjustment following a sudden emotional trauma? Thoughts and beliefs such as 'I will always feel the way that I do at this time', 'I will always think of past situations in the way that I do now' and 'There will never be anything that will change' will only serve to preserve negative beliefs about yourself and the stifle the prospect of these changing. What are your best hopes for how things could change? What strengths do you have that you might be overlooking?

Do you think about every situation or event in the exact same way every time that you think about it? If not, what might contribute to this? Is there any chance that you might allow this to happen here too, even if you currently cannot possibly imagine it? Because you have now allowed yourself to imagine what a new future might look like, are you perhaps equating this with there being no future? This may be possible when you summarize progress as proposed on page 109.

World

- Since Sarah died, I realize that the world is a bad place.
- The death of Sarah has made me realize that we live in an awful world.

- The death of Sarah has taught me that the world is unjust.
- The death of Sarah has taught me that the world is a worthless place.

Thinking in this way gives rise to a number of consequences, not to mention the prolongation of grief and a greater likelihood of feeling stuck. Engaging with life after your bereavement doesn't seem appealing as the world is viewed in such negative terms. This will also fuel the focus on loss and all the actions and responses that serve to maintain the separation and pain linked with complicated grief.

I have to preface this next section with the acknowledgement that of course some extremely tragic and awful events happen in life. The death of the person you have been close to may have happened as a result of crime, assault or a dreadful accident. Although we tend not to linger on the painful and distressing aspects of life, there are indeed times when it is full of despair, confusion, distress, pain and hurt. Some people experience this much more than others and unfortunately there seems to be no rhyme or reason to this – there isn't a rule that bad things should only happen once, or only to people who have been malicious or abusive to others; or that good things should be reserved to those who seem deserving of positive consequences. Viewing death as unfair and unjust is often the result of comparisons with other people where death would have seemed 'fairer' – for example, the death of a young child in a road traffic accident may well seem very unfair given that her grandmother has long been suffering a terminal illness and is 'ready to go'. The grandmother's death might have seemed 'fairer'.

These thoughts link with beliefs about order in the word, and perhaps a belief that people should not die at certain ages or that parents should always die before their children. Personal beliefs are often at odds with deaths: people who invest time and energy in health-promoting activity die suddenly or, conversely, people who abuse their bodies and take no interest in health promotion live beyond the expected lifespan, perhaps 'unfairly' given other people you may know who have died younger.

We do live in a world where awful things happen every day. There are thousands of deaths through accidents and murders. Some people do set out to harm and kill other people, and there are those who have to endure intolerable physical and mental torture at the hands of criminals intent on killing and maiming others. It is inevitable that, when your own world is so dominated by loss, separation and pain, these will come to crowd your mind. Changing these thoughts does not mean that these things will not happen.

The change in thinking can be subtle and the aim is to move from 'we live in an awful world' or 'the world is unjust' to a mindset that acknowledges that, while there are many things happening in the world that are not fair and that represent tragedy – and that these are of course accompanied by sadness and distress – they are not the complete picture. The hundreds of thousands of actions and outcomes that take place every day to enhance people's lives are much more prevalent and outnumber the sadness and loss considerably. What could be done to help restore your faith in the world? What solutions are within your control to make your world more positive, even if only slightly to start with?

Life

- Life has nothing to offer me any more.
- My life is useless since Sarah died.
- My life is meaningless since Sarah died.
- My life has no meaning any more, since Sarah died.

Thoughts about a life devoid of meaning are often associated with clinically significant depressive symptoms. If you have such thoughts and are feeling depressed and hopeless, with no enjoyment or pleasure in day-to-day activities, you should consider speaking with your doctor or practice nurse about the possibility that you are clinically depressed. You should also think about some of the activities and events that formerly provided a sense of meaning, particularly those that did not depend upon the person who has died. What would someone who loved you say if he or she knew you were thinking that life was meaningless? What would the person who died say? Is it possible that, even though you don't see any meaning at the moment, this is something that you could build into your life with some support and help? Are you comparing the level of meaning you had when life was going well with the level of meaning now, and concluding that because this is less there is none at all? What would need to be happening for life to have some meaning and how could you take a step towards this?

Future

- I don't expect that I will feel better in the future.
- I don't have confidence in the future.
- My wishes for the future will never be fulfilled.
- In the future I will never again be really happy.
- Since Sarah is no longer here, I have a negative view on the future.

The future will never be the same as before, and it could be that accepting this is the first step towards restoring aspects of life where you have some level of fulfilment and pleasure. Confidence is not something that will emerge until you can feel supported to take some small steps towards a new future – a future that is the unknown, where some days it will all feel overwhelming and the level of enthusiasm for living will not be a patch on what you have felt before. What happens if you allow your mind to consider a future with some respite from the pain of grief? Is there something that could be done to influence things for the better?

Self-blame

- I am partially responsible for Sarah's death.
- I should have prevented the death of Sarah.
- If I had done things differently, Sarah would still be alive.
- I will never be able to forgive myself for the things I did wrong in the relationship with Sarah.
- I blame myself for not having cared better for Sarah.

Carefully consider all the factors that contributed to the death of the person you are mourning. You could list them all and then, one by one, think about how much, in percentage terms, this contributed to the person's death. Did you put yourself on the list? Did you really contribute to the death? Did your care and decision-making contribute the major part of the events that caused the death? What would people who know you well say if you told them that you have contributed to the death?

Others

- The people around me should give me more support.
- Many people have let me down after Sarah's death.
- People around me should show much more interest in me.

Do other people know that you are thinking in this way? Could it be that they have good intentions but that, linked with the pain of loss and separation, you are feeling their absence more intently? What would happen if you took the step of saying to some people that you need support from them? It could be that they genuinely need assistance with thinking about your needs, and that when you ask for help they will gladly provide it to you. People may find it challenging to know what you need if you have not felt able to tell them. What first step could you take to reach out to other people to help them support you?

Appropriateness

- My grief reactions are abnormal.
- I don't mourn the way I should do.
- I do not react to this loss normally.
- There is something wrong with my feelings.

Does thinking about your reactions this way help you towards recovery? Have you learned anything in this book that might contradict this, or make you question whether in fact your reactions are as abnormal as you have thought? Who says that your reaction is not normal, that it should be different or that there is something wrong with the reactions? What could you say to yourself based on what you have learned that explains why your reactions are understandable? Could the model about healing help explain why your reactions are to be expected, and how the changes can start when you begin to confront some of the stuck points, to reverse some avoidance and begin to plan for the times when you can experience the pain and distress without the avoidance?

Cherishing grief

- I have to mourn, otherwise I will forget Sarah.
- As long as I mourn I maintain the bond with Sarah.
- As long as I mourn I do not really have to let Sarah go.

Would it help if you were to plan in a time when you will specifically mourn your loss – reassuring yourself that this can be a part of your life without it dominating all aspects of each day? The next chapters look at helping you to have a lasting memorial, incorporating pictures and memories, meaning that the loved one who is no longer here in person can still be a part of your life, and that the memories can become integrated with a range of other memories and experiences as you rebuild and restore your life.

Threatening interpretation of grief – fear of your feelings

- If I let go of my emotions, I will go crazy.
- If I fully realized what the death of Sarah means, I would go crazy.
- If I allowed my feelings to come out, I would lose control.
- If I once started crying, I would lose control.

Do you have images of losing control of your mind? Do you feel that your emotions have some quality that makes you fear they will spiral out of control? Are you perhaps holding on too much, avoiding so much that this is creating the fear that you will lose control? In fact, if you allow yourself to feel, it will be painful but, at the same time, connecting with the intense pain links you with the bond you have lost. It can also act as a trigger to ensure that you invest time and energy into remembering its legacy and impact on you and your life. If you can feel this emotion it can act as a reminder of the need to begin to rebuild and restore elements of your life. Would it help you to say to yourself that, if you take the feelings slowly and express them in a measured way at first, you will slowly gain some control over them?

It might be helpful to pay attention to the kind of words you are using when you talk or think about the impact of the death on your life. Look out in particular for words such as 'always', 'should' and 'can't'. These extremes of thinking can influence adjustment too, so if you notice them try to replace them with less extreme words.

You might be concluding something based on no evidence, or even when all the facts and information suggest an entirely different conclusion. If you are jumping to conclusions, spend some time thinking about any elements that, owing to the intensity of your distress, you have not considered. Even if this seems difficult and deep down you cannot see it as being possible, it will become easier to change your feelings if you can begin to think about this theoretically – in the way that you might point it out to someone else. When we are distressed we tend to exaggerate negative aspects of our experience and at the same time minimize (or shrink) information that could be vital in helping with adjustment to a situation.

Beliefs about loss and grief

The next section looks at the way in which your beliefs might have been affected by your experience of loss and grief. This might be easy to explain if you have a good awareness of it and/or have discussed it with other people. More usually, though, this thinking process is not so easy to put into words.

- What has happened since your loss that has had the most unsettling effect on you?
- What was the most disturbing aspect of this experience for you?
- Did it cause you to question something that you believed unconditionally or completely?
- What sort of issues about you, your life and the world in general have you had to grapple with mentally?

You will develop more insight and awareness into this as you move through some of the exercises in this book, so don't be too concerned if examples do not come to mind at this point. The important thing is the notion that your beliefs before the death will be reconsidered in light of the death as your mind attempts to make sense of what has happened.

Beliefs about death:

- Death is inevitable and need not be feared.
- Death can be a very positive force for changing perspectives.
- Death causes pain and heartache of the most powerful sort.

Beliefs about grief:

- Grief is all-consuming and needs to be respected.
- Grief can be shown in very many different ways.
- When I feel grief I tend to have peaks and troughs of crying.

A thought or belief can be assimilated into your overall way of thinking, but if it does not fit with this it needs to be accommodated. This is not an easy notion.

Accommodating beliefs about death

Acknowledging the permanence of the death, and having to readjust and reconstruct previously held thoughts and beliefs about the person who has died, about your own life pattern and about life in general, is tremendously difficult. It is often only when this has happened that readjustment of life goals and expectations can occur. Stuck points are often the result of an inability to fit events into a framework of thoughts – or assimilating them – or when other thoughts need to be developed in order to restore some sort of order or meaning to the overall view of the world – new thoughts are what develop when you accommodate the change resulting from grief.

Bereavement and death may result in you questioning prior beliefs about religion and mortality. This can lead to a 'spiritual crisis' where faith in God is brought into question, though for some people discovery of faith and spiritual dimensions of life occurs during the new life imposed by loss.

Cognitive Behavioural Therapy (CBT) is based on the premise that the use of questions can enable people to identify elements of their thoughts or experiences that are otherwise not linked or used to assist with coping with events or the emotional reactions to them. This model, applied to understanding grief, is based on the position that it is not grief that is linked with problem moods, thoughts or behaviours but the thoughts about grief and coping with it that are important. There are many related models that also propose a different approach to these thoughts, some viewing these as requiring practical solutions and others as something to accept without allowing them to dominate psychological wellbeing.

The death of an attachment figure means that there is a mismatch between the mental notion or memory of a loved one and the intellectual knowledge that they are dead. The power of the mental model means that the mental presence of the loved one as a significant attachment remains. The attachment system (which is hardwired into all of us) triggers attempts to bring you closer to the person – this is what causes the yearning and longing, and explains how the thoughts and memories of the person are generated in a bid to maintain closeness and connection with him or her. There is disruption in the processes that control attachment-seeking and links with the wider world – meaning that interest in the wider world is diminished and focus on goal attainment and planning is lessened. The level of interest in other people and in usual daily activities is much reduced during this acute grief response.

7

Using memories and the power of the mind to rebuild connections

This chapter looks at the way in which complicated grief tends to shut out a wider range of memories of the person who has died, serving to keep the emphasis on the pain and distress of grief. Thus, complicated grief can prevent you from accessing a wider range of information to help with adjusting to the loss, as well as with developing a fuller mental representation of the person, enriched by a wide range of memories based on all that you shared and that he or she meant to you.

Memories of the person who has died

In this next exercise you are encouraged to remember the dead person, allowing your mind to wander and flow freely. Don't be too concerned if initially your mind is overwhelmed with recent memories; note these down too. Remember to use the insights and tactics from earlier in this book if distress starts to overwhelm you. You may only be able to access other memories from other times in your life when you specifically use other techniques to bring them into your mind.

Exercise 7.1

See what memories come to mind, and jot them down in your notebook. Start with a very brief description of what the memory is (e.g. her smile when the baby took his first steps). When you have the memory fixed in your mind, expand on it by considering some of the questions below:

- When was this memory? Month and year?
- What do you remember about the person in this memory?
- Where was he or she in this memory?
- What was he or she doing? Was this typical?
- What other features of this memory make it special or one to note?

Remember that you can also include humorous anecdotes or happier memories if these come to mind. Don't be too concerned if this does not happen to start with; keep coming back to this exercise and discuss it with others. It may be that friends and family have memories of times when you and the person were together that they are happy to talk about. They may also have memories which, although not personally related to you, are memorable for other reasons. Don't feel disheartened if, the first few times you try this exercise, little or no information comes to mind. Keep focusing on it, and the memories will come in time.

Using pictures to support mourning

It is often painful to confront images (particularly video) of the person who has died, seeing them 'brought to life'. However, if you can face this, think of this phase in your recovery as a way of moving to a point where living without your loved one becomes tolerable – tolerable because you are able to actively remember, think, talk and focus on this person as part of your life.

You might not be able to face looking at pictures of the person who has died, especially in the first few months after the death. Looking at pictures is often very upsetting, particularly if you have tended to look at them occasionally or tentatively. In some extreme examples, people have not looked at any pictures of the person who has died. This was the case with one lady who attended my clinic. The first time she faced this was with my support in a consulting room at the hospital building. Her emotion was extremely intense, triggering thoughts that she would go 'crazy' and would suffocate with the pressure on her chest from the anxiety of seeing a picture of her husband laughing.

Pictures themselves can be ordered in a sequence according to the time they are associated with or, if some are more distressing, in accordance with the distress experienced. You will quickly know this if you see a picture and then have a strong urge to turn it over so that you do not have to face it.

Exercises in this book have focused on bringing memories to mind – in your thinking and writing, and maybe when you speak with your support network. Photos bring special, often painful memories of their very own but play an important part in helping people assimilate their grief.

Exercise 7.2

When you look at pictures to start with, your reactions will be very much as with all other reminders when grief has become complicated. Look through pictures and pay attention to your reactions, writing them down in your notebook.

The aim of this exercise is to expand your thinking, so that you can access a fuller range of memories about the person that includes happier times as well as the distressing run-up to the death and the way it happened. There will be things that you will always remember about your loved one, and among all your memories there will usually be especially cherished or favourite memories. As you begin to look at pictures and build up a more detailed summary of key memories, make a note beside those you feel are the special ones; you'll want to expand on this as part of acknowledging special times and meaningful links with the person who is no longer a living part of your life.

Make a personal commitment to use the pictures in the future as a source of comfort and benefit, evidence of how your life has been enhanced and enriched by having known the person who has died. You may not think about it in this way at the moment, though keeping it in your mind will help you focus on it as the aim of the work that is outlined in this chapter. One of the people I have worked with on this wrote: 'The complications with my grief make it hard for me to see that one day I will be able to experience some positive feelings – remembering how I have felt with Steven in the past will come to me as the pain eases.'

Another person was very frightened about what would happen to her levels of distress if she were to spend some time looking at pictures of her son who had died. She decided to write down a plan, including an element of 'reward' and support at the end –a general and important point for when you are planning elements of your recovery that involve more directly confronting the loss that you have experienced.

Plan: I will gather some of the photograph albums and put them all in the spare room on the bed. I will take one of them out and see what happens, see how I feel. I will do this on Monday afternoon at 3 p.m.

What happened? I felt that I was going to be sick with nerves as I had not looked at these for nearly a year.

What will I plan next? I will take a couple of them through to the other room, where I feel more relaxed and at home, and look at them there tomorrow afternoon at the same time. I think I will call Mary and ask if her if she wants to come round for a coffee about 4 p.m. tomorrow.

Choose a time when you will start to look through your pictures of the person who has died. You may start to feel anxious or apprehensive about this as the time approaches. Experiencing and expressing intense grief and emotion is not a pleasant experience, though this will be an important part of connecting with the feelings that are part of living your life now and understanding the most painful aspects of your grief experiences. It is only by fully focusing on these feelings that you will be able to confront the loss.

Sometimes you may not be sure if the person is in a particular picture, or you will not have looked at the pictures for some time. If you feel less apprehensive about seeing a picture that holds special meaning, you can spend some time with a friend, describing what is in the pictures as a way of introducing this to your plans for addressing your complicated grief reactions.

Make a point of noting down any emotions, thoughts and reactions when you are looking at the pictures. These could give some important clues about any points where you are struggling or stuck, as well as providing information that you can use in identifying the way in which the person who has died has influenced your life for the better – so this can be used as part of the planning for the future. Looking at pictures is painful, but it is a crucial part of helping you develop ways of living in a world where the person is no longer present. You might want to get some copies of these pictures made for other people; when you have been able to start looking at the pictures, providing copies to others and linking this with personally meaningful written words or items of personal significance can be part of linking your grief with a message or legacy to be passed on to others. Including some of these in boxes of memories can be therapeutic for some people.

When you can spend more time looking at the pictures and the emotions are less overwhelming and distressing for you, maybe consider the following:

- Do these photos remind you of times you have not been as aware of recently, or have half-forgotten? Is it possible for you to remember what these happier times felt like?
- Are there memories of events shared?
- Is there a shared experience that you feel sums up the person who is no longer here?
- Can this be expressed in words?
- What are the words that sum up the meanings and values you have identified in the pictures?

Exercise 7.3

Take some space in your notebook to write some notes on how you have used pictures and what you have noticed about your feelings as you spend more time looking at them, but also in terms of what memories, thoughts and experiences come more into your mind.

Now that you have chosen a set of pictures that signify the events that are most memorable or those that are personally significant because of what they illustrate to you about the person, think about what you would like to do with them.

You have focused on them and extracted information on their personal meaning as part of addressing the complications with your grief, but there may be other things that you would like to do with them. Do you want them to be on show? Are there people you might want to make copies for? You might want to arrange them in albums that are specifically designed for you to link with other work suggested in this book. As well as photos, an album might include your summary of the way in which you have changed some of your thinking and reactions to the death, with the summary statements and discoveries that you have noted from other sections of this book.

Research on adjustment to trauma has shown that resolving this in psychological terms often requires integration (joining up) of disparate information into a revised framework linking all the various emotions, memories and related thoughts into one whole.

This is a unique process and one that only you will understand. It has been described nicely by Dr Katherine Shear, who stated that 'when integration is accomplished, it is as though the deceased releases her grip on the mind of the mourner, in order to reside quietly in his heart. Yet this process can be arduous, proceeding in fits and starts' (Shear et al. 2007).

Now that you have spent some time focusing on the power of pictures and images, you have learned another useful element of restoring your links with the person who has died. This is a way of focusing on your grief when you want to, but also a way of reminding yourself of the connections, personal links and significance of the way in which this person has touched your life forever.

Using your imagination

In the same way that pictures can provide a way of expressing emotion and a framework for grief recovery, so too can beginning to use your imagination to make sense of unresolved thoughts or elements of personal impact. The next section outlines how to begin to use imagination as a new tactic in your increasing repertoire of skills. It can help to think about having an imaginary conversation with the person who has died. Begin by thinking that you are with the person who has died at the moment of death, and then focus on all the things that you have wanted to tell him or her.

Imagine that you are with the person just shortly after he or she has died. Now note down some of the things that you will say to them. When you have done this, spend some time on your own and talk 'with' the person; some people prefer to do this internally in their heads, though it is more effective if spoken out loud. Use your support person for this if that would be easier.

When you have done this, spend some time writing down all the points that you brought up in this talk, and then take on the role of the person who has died. Respond to each of the points that you made in speaking 'with' them. When you first start to do this, you will have only what you say written down:

Sarah, I can't believe that it has come to this. I feel so bereft – I can't stand it that you have gone.

I will never know such joy and laughter again. I wish I had made more of the good times, focused more on how precious life can be.

You looked so sore and weary. I should have done more but I have been beside myself with anxiety. Sorry.

Then some possible responses can be added in. These are shown in italics below, to illustrate how the responses are added after your record of the first section of the exercise.

Sarah, I can't believe that it has come to this. I feel so bereft – I can't stand it that you have gone.

I can't believe I am not near you in person. I am with you, though – I will never leave you, I am all around you.

I will never know such joy and laughter again. I wish I had made more of the good times, focused more on how precious life can be.

I know, my love, we won't ever laugh in life again – I remember all the times we did and it makes me smile. All the good times were vivid in my mind even when I was in pain.

You looked so sore and weary. I should have done more but I have been beside myself with anxiety. Sorry.

I was tired but your presence made me feel at ease. I know that people will be there for you. I want your anxiety to ease just as my tiredness has gone now. I am at peace and I want you to be too now.

It is important for you to allow positive memories to come into your mind about the person who has died, paying attention to this while you work on the conversation and capturing and noticing these as part of the aim of creating a rich set of mental connections to all the links with the person's life and what the two of you shared.

It may be helpful for you to focus on the years that you knew the person who has died, and to use this as a way of structuring what you record as you consider information about memories and events you shared when he or she was alive.

For example, if the person died when 55 years old and you met when he or she was 20 years old, you could structure this as follows:

20–30 years   The trip to London, the weekend lie-ins, when the boys were born

31–40 years	The laughs on our monthly night out at the pictures, the caring when I was ill
41–50 years	The walks at the weekend, the fun at Chelsea, conversations between the four of us
51–55 years	The contentment with our routine.

Keep coming back to the task over several days, adding new memories. When you eventually have a list of memories of events involving the person, this can be used to extract information about the personal significance of the memories. What does this memory tell you about the person? What does it say about his or her approach to life? How did this make you feel at the time? When you think about this memory now, what is the main feeling that you have? How could you extract details from this to inform a summary of the positive influence on your life that came as a result of knowing this person? Might there be other ways in which you could restore links with this legacy by planning future actions that would result in similar benefits? If you are unable to contemplate this just now, don't worry: this is something that will come to you as you start to focus more on how to cope with the loss and restore positive feelings in some aspects of your day-to-day life.

It is all right for you to bring negative memories into your mind, as the aim here is to remember the real person. The focus of memories in this way means that you can begin to recall the living person in all dimensions. This helps to give rise to a sense of connectedness with the person who has died in a completely different way from that which has been part of your current way of thinking.

Putting this all together

Take all the pictures and materials that you have gathered, including the imaginary conversation and your written summary of memories, and collect them together in one place. This in itself is likely to be distressing, and you should build in some way of being able to take yourself out of the task, pausing or telling someone that you are planning to do it and arranging for support while you do so.

Helen told her best friend, Sheena, that she was planning to spend some time in the afternoon looking through her late husband's chest of drawers and selecting items of clothing that could be donated to charity. Helen knew that doing this would require access to other memories of her husband, beyond those that were uppermost in her mind and/or related to the immediate recent past, and that this could have therapeutic value in relation to increased availability in memory of events that had been shared or information about her husband from happier times.

Helen asked Sheena to call round a couple of hours afterwards, so that she knew she would have her support if she needed it and could talk to her about how it had been. Sheena was pleased to have been asked to assist.

How might this apply to your coping plan? There could be trigger events or tasks that would be easier to deal with if you were to plan for something to happen after the task has been started or when there has been a trigger event or action. You could take a similar approach to times when you are planning work outlined in this book, scheduling tasks and/or a supportive visit from a friend around the time that you are planning to work on these topics.

8

Creating a lasting memorial

The need for a memorial to mark a death has long been recognized as an important element of adjusting to death and coping with bereavement. The therapeutic benefits of investing time in establishing a memorial as a means of expressing emotion, acknowledging the meaning of the deceased person's life and death and mobilizing interpersonal support will be outlined in this chapter. The creation of a lasting memorial is something that you can build on when you have made progress with confronting distress, understanding thoughts, reversing avoidance and making sense of the way that memories and links with the person can become an integral part of a life restored.

As you have worked through this book, you have spent some time focusing on memories of the person who has died, thinking about the way in which he or she has influenced your life and how his or her death has impacted upon your views about yourself, the world and the people around you. Now you may want to think about how to capture some of the most meaningful elements in a memorial.

This is a term that is often associated with a public gesture. However, although this can be an element of your plans, memorials can also be very private and personal arrangements with particular significance only to those close to the person who has died. In some cases, you may wish arrange for something to happen in memory of the person – a special event or gesture that signifies the importance of that person's life and death to you.

In thinking about this, you may find it helpful to think about what you would want other people to know about your loved one. Is there something about his life and the manner in which he died that you would like to share with other people? Are there elements of her approach to life and living that other people may not have appreciated, or that if they did know about could make a positive contribution to their life and approach to living? What elements of the memorial would help with your adjustment now and as you move into the future?

As you work on creating a memorial, it is important to keep track of the way in which you have been reacting to the idea of a memorial emotionally, both within your thinking and in the way you are relating to other people and life in general. This can provide a balance between focusing on the losses and grief that you have experienced and providing an outlet and bridge to the future. Hopefully, it will reflect some of the work that you have undertaken in relation to being able to recount the details of the circumstances leading to the death, the subsequent events (even if only in a brief form to provide context), the personal impact on you and how, through support and taking time to consider all that the person has meant to you, your life has been changed and will continue to be influenced by him or her in the future.

Where do you begin?

If you don't know where to begin in planning this, then here are some initial pointers to help you:

- Name of the person who died
- Date of birth and date of death
- Brief details of the circumstances of his or her death
- Some notes on the person and his or her life
- Some notes on the person's contribution to life, meaning to you and other people
- A description of what you see as the person's legacy.

Review the notes and details that you have written in your notebook as you have worked through the other chapters, to see if this helps with your notes in planning a memorial. You might want to look at obituaries published in newspapers or online, to give you ideas of ways of communicating what someone has meant to you. Phrases or wording that others have used will give you examples or ideas of what you might wish to incorporate into your lasting memorial. Some people choose to commit to participating in a sporting endeavour or personal challenge, linking this with fund-raising for a charity that is related to the person who died.

Other issues can also be part of creating a memorial. The planning and discussion for this can begin to provide a purpose and could even be the way that previously avoided activities are reintroduced into daily living, though in a way that is still connected with mourning. Look through the pictures you have collected, speak to colleagues, family members and friends, and think about these questions:

- Did the person have a favourite place?
- Is this somewhere that you visited together?
- If you look back on the person's life, what is the most important element of his or her approach for you?
- What do you want to remember most of all about his or her death (including the impact of the death)?
- What are the main elements of the way in which the person adjusted to illness?
- What was his or her philosophy for living? Perhaps this inspired you and you would like to be able to incorporate elements of this into your life.

Think about how you would like to feel when the memorial is in place – what would be the most helpful aspect for you personally? Remember that you are the one who can control and influence this, so take time to plan and contemplate how this can work best for you in supporting your recovery. Would you want this memorial to be publicly acknowledged, or would you prefer it to be anonymous, known about only by you and those you chose to tell that the memorial is there?

This need not involve visiting a cemetery or tending a grave, though for many people this helps them feel closer to the person who has died. Others can achieve this level of connection without leaving their home or through symbolic aspects of other memorials that are created. The memorial might be as simple as a small ornament or a section of a display cabinet with a photograph and something personal that was important or belonged to the person. There are infinite possibilities, the only constraints being how to generate ideas and bring them to fruition.

Memorials following the death of a loved one might traditionally be thought of in terms of the headstones and marble tributes that adorn cemeteries and gardens of remembrance. These are of course hugely significant elements of remembering the life and legacy of someone who has died, though if you start to generate ideas and alternatives you will quickly appreciate that there are several ways in which it is possible to remember someone.

Some people might embark upon a trip or journey intended to celebrate or honour the memory of a person or an event, particularly if this involves visiting places of personal significance to the person who has died, or perhaps places that you shared together. Doing this acknowledges the reality of the loss, but also provides a continuing sense of connection with your loved one that is such an important part of adjusting to life without him or her. It also helps with the creation of new memories that are based on the trip, building a body of information about how the person's legacy and meaning to you are a positive influence for good in your life now. You may want to visit places you shared with the person or, having identified issues that have personal meaning, visit places linked with that.

In some cases, a written statement of facts or a petition presented to a legislative body or an executive could be progressed in memory of someone who has died, particularly if that person's death has been contributed to by factors that require public sector improvements, legislative change or societal call to action. This is the case when deaths occur as a result of accidents or avoidable systems failures such as sometimes occur in the healthcare or other service industry. It may be worth considering establishing an award or charity link.

A memorial serves to remember someone, commemorating that person's life and marking his or her death. I have often thought that, particularly for sudden deaths, societal requirements for burial and the intense distress that can accompany the shock of a death make it more difficult to develop a memorial that takes account of all the aspects that one might wish to include – the pain and acute nature of grief can make this difficult. This is not to say that it will not be difficult at other times, though the point here is that memorial acts are likely to be more helpful and comprehensive and less influenced by the acute pain of grief if they are planned and enacted several weeks after the death has occurred.

In some cases people themselves may have expressed a view of how they wish this to be actioned, particularly if they have been involved in planning events after their death – perhaps as part of end-of-life care planning in the context of palliative care for a progressive and incurable disease.

The memorial can become something that is associated with emotional expression, as well as a way of communicating more widely about the legacy, meaning and impact of the person who has died. The proliferation of technology, social media sites and globalization has resulted in a wider range of options and more accessibility in creating memorials for people. There are also an increasing number of companies that focus on supporting and enabling people to create memorials through audiovisual media.

You may want to think about looking at the memorials that other people have created for their loved ones, visiting these, gathering pictures, information and poems and then taking some time to create something of your own. In some cases you may never share this and it becomes something that is for personal reflection and use only. Some of the ideas are outlined below; you can add to these as you consider and reflect on possible additional ideas for your planning and actions.

Ideas for a memorial

- Plant a tree, shrub or bush in a garden (which could be accompanied with an external sign to signify what it commemorates).
- Collect photographs of the person and file these with an album that has been specifically bought for this purpose.
- Have a star named after the person who has died (there are many companies offering this online).
- Collect together some music, pictures and video on to one source such as a DVD for review.
- Choose a significant image or picture, or have this commissioned by a professional artist.
- Make a donation or carry out some work or fundraising activity in your loved one's name.

- Adopt an animal or sponsor a child as part of a charity-giving programme.
- Make a selection of key verse and poems.
- Create a website or 'space' on the web.
- Create a book of remembrance (online or in actual print).

People are of course different with respect to what they would find helpful or meaningful. We all have different preferences in terms of the written word, pictures, music, film, places and approach. It may even be that the way in which you would find it helpful to develop a memorial would not be something that would have been appreciated by the person who has died. One of the key certainties is that this is a very personal decision that will need to balance the preferences of the person who has died with those of the people who have been most affected by the death.

You may not necessarily be thinking about the personal psychological benefits at the time (as thoughts are often outwardly focused on the activity itself or on the linkages between why you are doing the event and the death of the person). However, these sorts of memorial activities are a vital part of restoring and investing in your life and in the way in which you live, understand and engage with it and understand the impact of death. They can serve as a public communication that you have reached a point where you are ready to acknowledge the reality of the loss and that things will continue, firmly and clearly marking the person's life – and also death – as a part of your remaining years. They are something to be acknowledged and integrated into the time you have left (as opposed to forgotten and avoided as a reminder only of the past).

Memorials can then become part of a developing network of memories and experiences. Decisions that are made will become part of your own life history and associated with conversations, links and other memories within new relationships and experiences. You can remember the person who has died in ways that only you are aware of – indeed, simply bringing him or her to mind and/or recalling a specific memory of a shared experience is in itself a memorial to your lost loved one.

9

Life will never be the same

Grief can be thought of as integrated when the final nature of the death has been acknowledged and the consequences of this for life have also been acknowledged and evaluated. Thoughts and memories concerning the person who has died have been ordered and revised to take account of the death in a way that allows for life goals to be clarified and implemented.

Do not to be too concerned if some of the things that helped you yesterday, last week or last month are less helpful today. This does not mean that they will not be helpful again. There will be different factors influencing the way that you are thinking and feeling, emotionally and physically, and there might need to be a different solution today.

Take some time to review all the exercises you have completed in this book and think about how you can pay attention to the changes you have made, focus on new things, feel distracted from your grief and invest time in thinking about new ways of living your life. Think about what you have learned about the impact of grief on your life and the ways in which you are more able to experience the anguish, knowing that the intensity of the pain passes if you can express it and link it with details of the way in which your life was enriched and enhanced by the person who has died. When you have done this, try to summarize it in your notebook. It may help to start like this:

> Although my life will never be the same, I have learned through understanding the complicated nature of grief that . . .

Carefully re-read the summary of the events surrounding the death and think about how you see this now. Notice any changes in emotion, approach and perspective. These are the building blocks of restoring your quality of life and wellbeing. You may find that as this happens you notice yourself having other reactions, or that new thoughts start to emerge within your consciousness; these could be thoughts about the past or ways in which your current and future life might be impacted by what has happened. Write these down too.

Now think about the pictures, the imaginary conversation that you have developed and the memorial in place for the person who has died. If you could sum all this up, how would you do it? Think about how your life has been changed because of the person, how the rest of your life will be influenced by his or her death and how you can live your life in a way that not only acknowledges the pain and distress of the loss but tries to channel this into something that strengthens you, perhaps by re-creating experiences that remind you of how you felt when you were with your loved one, perhaps visiting places or having experiences that remind you of past times. Add this to your summary.

And finally, there may be several areas where you are still concerned or troubled about your grief reactions. Remember that it is possible you may need to use some of the techniques again – focusing on memories of what happened, reducing avoidance of this and improving the connections in your memory, focusing on the way in which your thoughts have sticking points or you have been unable to move memories from your mind to your heart. If this does not help then think about speaking with a healthcare professional or support person to consider more ways to help with your recovery.

I hope that this book has helped you understand more about how you have reacted to significant death or loss in your life and that, by applying some of the ideas and reflecting on the issues and questions raised, you have been helped in restoring some of the natural psychological healing mechanisms that became blocked and caused your grief to be complicated. Where complications have occurred, I hope you have been able to identify them and, through slowly confronting them and identifying ways of coping that help you to contain distress, will be able to confront them without fear. Use this to strengthen your resolve to live the rest of your life with a clear understanding of what your loss has meant to you, memories that you can use to build a happier future and plans to restore your sense of the world to one that is less distressing and dominated by grief.

References and further reading

Boelen, P. A. and Prigerson, H. G. (2007) 'The influence of symptoms of prolonged grief disorder, depression, and anxiety on quality of life among bereaved adults', *European Archives of Psychiatry and Clinical Neuroscience* 257(8): 444–52.

Hayes, Steven C. and Wilson, Kelly G. (2003) 'Mindfulness: method and process', *Clinical Psychology: Science and Practice* 10(2): 161–5.

Malkinson, R. (2010) 'Cognitive–behavioral grief therapy: the ABC model of Rational–Emotion Behavior Therapy', *Psihologijske teme* 19(2): 289–305.

Meert, K. L., Donaldson, A. E., Newth, C. J. L., Harrison, R., Berger, J., Zimmerman, J., Anand, K. J. S., Carcillo, J., Dean, J. M. and Willson, D. F. (2010) 'Complicated grief and associated risk factors among parents following a child's death in the pediatric intensive care unit', *Archives of Pediatrics and Adolescent Medicine* 164(11): 1045–51.

Parkes, C. M. (1998) 'Coping with loss: bereavement in adult life', *British Medical Journal* 316(7134): 856–9.

Shear, M. K. (2010) 'Exploring the role of experiential avoidance from the perspective of attachment theory and the dual process model', *OMEGA – Journal of Death and Dying* 61(4): 357–69.

Shear, M. K. and Mulhare, E. (2008) 'Complicated grief', *Psychiatric Annals* 38(10): 662–70.

Shear, M. K. and Shair, H. (2005) 'Attachment, loss, and complicated grief', *Developmental Psychobiology* 47(3): 253–67.

Shear, M. K., Frank, E., Houck, P. R. and Reynolds, C. F. III (2005) 'Treatment of complicated grief', *JAMA: The Journal of the American Medical Association* 293(21): 2601–8.

Shear, M. K., Jackson, C., Essock, S., Donahue, S. and Felton, C. (2006) 'Screening for complicated grief among Project Liberty service recipients 18 months after September 11, 2001', *Psychiatric Services* 57(9): 1291–7.

Shear, M. K., Monk, T., Houck, P., Melhem, N., Frank, E., Reynolds, C. and Sillowash, R. (2007) 'An attachment-based model of complicated grief including the role of avoidance', *European Archives of Psychiatry and Clinical Neuroscience* 257(8): 453–61.

Stroebe, M. and Schut, H. (1999) 'The dual process model of coping with bereavement: rationale and description', *Death Studies* 23(3): 197–224.

Stroebe, M. and Schut, H. (2010) 'The dual process model of coping with bereavement: a decade on', *OMEGA – Journal of Death and Dying* 61(4): 273–89.

Index